Primary HIV Infection – Pathology, Diagnosis, Management

Edited by Heiko Jessen and Hans Jaeger

26 Figures
12 Tables

Georg Thieme Verlag
Stuttgart · New York

Bibliographic Information published by
Die Deutsche Bibliothek

Die Deutsche Bibliothek lists this publication
in the Deutsche Nationalbibliografie;
detailed bibliographic data is available on
the internet at http://dnb.ddb.de.

© 2005 Georg Thieme Verlag KG
Rüdigerstraße 14
70469 Stuttgart, Germany
http://www.thieme.de
Thieme New York, 333 Seventh Avenue
New York, NY 10001, USA
http://www.thieme.com

Printed in Germany

Cover design by Thieme Verlagsgruppe
Cover photo: PhotoDisc, Inc.
Figures by Ziegler + Müller, Kirchentellinsfurt
Typesetting by Ziegler + Müller, Kirchentellinsfurt
Printing and Bookbinding by Grafisches Centrum
   Cuno GmbH & Co. KG, Calbe

ISBN 3-13-133541-6 (GTV)
ISBN 1-58890-416-4 (TNY)

1 2 3 4 5 6

To Marla

Foreword

In the first European PHI Symposium – EPHIS – in Berlin, Germany, we were able to bring together leading immunologists, virologists, and clinicians to present and discuss their most recent results of Primary HIV-1 Infection (PHI) research. The symposium was held under the patronage of Klaus Wowereit, the Governing Mayor of Berlin. The present publication contains summaries of the presentations and proceedings of the symposium, as well as recent expert opinions.

The need for such a meeting is owed to the particular importance of the early HIV infection phase for the course of the epidemic. Pilot studies suggest that treatment at the very early stages can dramatically alter the course of the infection. This offers a chance to reduce the risks associated with long-term treatment, in particular the development of resistance to therapy. Furthermore, some authors of this publication assume that up to 50% of all new HIV infections could be caused by acutely infected patients, due to their extremely high viral load. But only 10 to 25% of all PHI patients are identified by their physicians. Here, increased medical training focussing on primary HIV infection is vital.

We need to better understand the complexities of the pathogenesis and the options available to influence it. Can early treatment enhance an effective immune response? What is the impact of immune-based interventions? Answers to such fundamental questions are crucial and could possibly advance the development of therapeutic or preventative vaccines – perhaps the only prospect for overcoming this medical and humanitarian crisis.

We thank all the participants and authors for their dedication and commitment and are very grateful to everyone who contributed to the organisation of the event. In particular, we would like to thank Mr. Hendrik Streeck for his tireless work on the logistics and Dr. Arne B. Jessen for his valuable overall assistance. Without the generous support of Abbott Virology this publication and indeed the EPHIS symposium itself would not have been possible. Specifically we would like to express our gratitude to Dr. Dörte Kurz and Mr. Oliver Rauch of Abbott Virology.

We hope that the symposium has inspired numerous debates on this important aspect of the pandemic and contributed to the combat against it. In this spirit we are looking forward to the next EPHIS meeting.

Berlin and Munich,
July 2005

Heiko Jessen
Hans Jaeger

Addresses

Editors

Heiko Jessen, MD
Gemeinschaftspraxis Heiko Jessen
and Arne B. Jessen, MD,
Motzstr. 19,
10777 Berlin, Germany
E-mail: mail@praxis-jessen.de

Hans Jaeger, MD,
Karlsplatz/Stachus 8,
80335 Munich, Germany
E-mail: info@jajaprax.de

Authors

Todd M. Allen, PhD
Partners AIDS Research Center
and Infectious Disease Division,
Massachusetts General Hospital
and Harvard Medical School,
Boston, MA 02114, USA
E-mail: tallen2@partners.org

Marcus Altfeld, MD, PhD
Partners AIDS Research Center
and Infectious Disease Division,
Massachusetts General Hospital,
149 13th Street,
Boston, MA 02129, USA
E-mail: maltfeld@partners.org

Charles A. B. Boucher, PD, MD
UMC Utrecht, G04.614,
Heidelberglaan 100,
3584 CX Utrecht, The Netherlands
E-mail: C.Boucher@azu.nl

Edmée C. Bowles, MD
UMC Utrecht, G04.614,
Heidelberglaan 100,
3584 CX Utrecht, The Netherlands
E-mail: E.C.Bowles@azu.nl

David A. Cooper, MD, DSc
National Centre in HIV Epidemiology
and Clinical Research,
University of New South Wales,
376 Victoria Street,
Sydney, NSW 2010, Australia
E-mail: Dcooper@nchecr.unsw.edu.au

Sean Emery, PhD
Therapeutic and Vaccine Research Program,
National Centre in HIV Epidemiology
and Clinical Research,
University of New South Wales,
376 Victoria Street,
Sydney, NSW 2010, Australia
E-mail: semery@nchecr.unsw.edu.au

Matthias Freiwald, MD
Private Clinic,
Fuggerstr. 19,
10777 Berlin, Germany
E-mail: info@freiwald-rausch.de

Jörg Gölz, MD
DAGNAE e. V.,
Blondelstr. 9,
52062 Aachen, Germany
E-mail: verein@dagnae.de

Armin Goetzenich
DAGNAE e. V.,
Blondelstr. 9,
52062 Aachen, Germany
E-mail: verein@dagnae.de

Alexandre Harari
Laboratory of AIDS Immunopathogenesis,
Division of Immunology and Allergy,
Department of Medicine,
Centre Hospitalier Universitaire Vaudois,
University of Lausanne, 1011 Lausanne,
Switzerland
E-mail: Alexandre.Harari@chuv.ch

Hans Jaeger, MD
KIS-Curatorium for Immunodeficiency,
Munich, Germany
Karlsplatz/Stachus 8,
80335 Munich, Germany
E-mail: info@jajaprax.de

Heiko Jessen, MD
Gemeinschaftspraxis Heiko Jessen
and Arne B. Jessen, MD,
Motzstr. 19,
10777 Berlin, Germany
E-mail: mail@praxis-jessen.de

Daniel E. Kaufmann, MD
Partners AIDS Research Center
and Infectious Disease Division,
Massachusetts General Hospital,
149 13th Street,
Boston, MA 02129, USA
E-mail: dkaufmann@partner.org

Anthony D. Kelleher, MD, PhD
Immunovirology Laboratory Program,
Centre for Immunology, National Centre
in HIV Epidemiology and Clinical Research,
Cnr of West and Boundary Streets,
Darlinghurst, NSW 2010, Australia
E-mail: t.kelleher@cfi.unsw.edu.au

Laurene M. Kelly, MS
Research Institute for Genetic and Human Therapy
(RIGHT) at IRCCS Policlinico S. Matteo,
P. le Golgi 2,
27100 Pavia, Italy
and Washington, DC, USA
E-mail: rightpv@tin.it

Heribert Knechten, MD
DAGNAE e. V.,
Blondelstr. 9,
52062 Aachen, Germany
E-mail: verein@dagnae.de

Christine Kögl, PhD
MUC Research GmbH,
Karlsplatz 8,
80335 Munich, Germany
E-mail: cko@mucresearch.de

Mathias Lichterfeld
Partners AIDS Research Center
and Infectious Disease Division,
Massachusetts General Hospital,
149 13th Street,
Boston, MA 02129, USA
E-mail: mlichterfeld@partners.org

Julianna Lisziewicz, PhD
Research Institute for Genetic and Human Therapy
(RIGHT) at IRCCS Policlinico S. Matteo,
P. le Golgi 2,
27100 Pavia, Italy
and Washington, DC, USA
E-mail: rightpv@tin.it

Franco Lori, MD
Research Institute for Genetic and Human Therapy
(RIGHT) at IRCCS Policlinico S. Matteo,
P. le Golgi 2,
27100 Pavia, Italy
and Washington, DC, USA
E-mail: rightpv@tin.it

Giuseppe Pantaleo, MD
Laboratory of AIDS Immunopathogenesis,
Division of Immunology and Allergy,
Department of Medicine, Centre Hospitalier
Universitaire Vaudois, University of Lausanne,
1011 Lausanne, Switzerland
E-mail: giuseppe.pantaleo@chuv.ch

Timothy P. T. Ramacciotti, MD
Primary Infection Unit, National Centre in
HIV Epidemiology and Clinical Research,
University of New South Wales,
376 Victoria Street,
Sydney, NSW 2010, Australia
E-mail: tramacciotti@nchecr.unsw.edu.au

Knud Schewe, MD
Private Clinic St. Georg,
Brennerstr. 71,
20099 Hamburg, Germany
E-mail: schewe@praxis-st-georg.de

Don E. Smith, MD
Primary Infection Unit, National Centre in
HIV Epidemiology and Clinical Research,
University of New South Wales,
376 Victoria Street,
Sydney, NSW 2010, Australia
E-mail: dsmith@nchecr.unsw.edu.au

Giuseppe Tambussi, MD
Clinic of Infectious Diseases,
San Raffaele Scientific Institute,
20132 Milano, Italy
E-mail: g.tambussi@hrs.it

Joerg Timm, MD
Partners AIDS Research Center and
Infectious Disease Division, Massachusetts
General Hospital and Harvard Medical School,
Boston, Massachusetts 02114, USA
E-mail: jtimm@partners.org

Bruce D. Walker, MD
Partners AIDS Research Center and
Infectious Disease Division,
Massachusetts General Hospital,
149 13th Street,
Boston, MA 02129, USA
E-mail: bwalker@partners.org

Eva Wolf, PhD
MUC Research GmbH,
Karlsplatz 8,
80335 Munich, Germany
E-mail: info@jajaprax.de

Table of Contents

1 Pathology 1

1.1 Functional Characterization
of HIV-1-Specific CD4 T Cells 1
A. Harari, G. Pantaleo

1.2 Immunodominance of HIV-1-Specific
CD8$^+$ T Cell Responses in Acute
HIV-1 Infection 5
M. Lichterfeld, M. Altfeld

1.3 Impact of Viral Sequence Evolution
on Immune Control of HIV-1 12
J. Timm, T. M. Allen

2 New Approaches 21

2.1 Immune-Based Therapies in the
Treatment of HIV/AIDS 21
L. M. Kelly, J. Lisziewicz, F. Lori

2.2 Long-Term Control of HIV-1 RNA
Replication Following a Unique STI
and Mycophenolate Mofetil Therapy in
Patients Treated with HAART Since PHI 32
G. Tambussi

2.3 Supervised Treatment Interruptions
in Acute HIV Infection 36
D. E. Kaufmann, B. D. Walker

2.4 Therapeutic Vaccination in PHI 44
*T. P. T. Ramacciotti, D. E. Smith, S. Emery,
A. D. Kelleher, D. A. Cooper*

3 Clinical Epidemiology and Management 60

3.1 Drug Resistance and Transmission
of Resistance 60
E. C. Bowles, C. A. B. Boucher

3.2 Management of Primary HIV Infection
in Germany. Preliminary Data from
Two German Cohorts 69
*C. Kögl, E. Wolf, A. Goetzenich,
H. Jessen, K. Schewe, M. Freiwald,
J. Goelz, H. Knechten, H. Jaeger*

3.3 Primary HIV Type 1 Infection 78
H. Jessen

Index 81

1 Pathology

1.1 Functional Characterization of HIV-1-Specific CD4 T Cells

A. Harari, G. Pantaleo

Primary HIV-1 infection is associated with an acute viral syndrome in about 40 – 90% of cases (Kahn and Walker, 1998). In addition, primary HIV-1 infection is also associated with high titers of HIV-1 replication and with a vigorous antiviral response. A major feature of primary HIV-1 infection is the extensive immune activation. During this period, activated and proliferating CD4 T cells support massive HIV-1 replication and production. The resulting dissemination of HIV-1 results in virus replication which then triggers an effector immune response.

CD4 T cells play a fundamental role in the generation of antigen-specific immune responses, and studies performed in mice have demonstrated that stimulation and expansion of antigen-specific CD4 T cells precedes that of CD8 T cells during acute virus infection *in vivo*. CD4 T cells do not seem to be critical for the generation of the primary virus-specific CD8 T cell response but rather for the maintenance of the CD8 T cell response over time during the chronic phase of the infection.

Primary HIV-1 infection is associated with a major oligoclonal expansion of HIV-1-specific CD8 T cells which generally coincides with the peak in viremia and precedes the neutralizing antibody response. The appearance of the cytotoxic T cells (CTL) response is temporally associated with the down-regulation of the viremia. This observation indicated a role for HIV-1-specific CD8 T cells in the initial control of virus replication. However, the direct demonstration of the key role played by CD8 T cells in the early control of the virus comes from the monkey SIV model. In fact, it has been demonstrated that the depletion of CD8 T cells resulted in a failure to control the initial peak of viremia in the infected animals.

Antibodies and cytotoxic CD8 T cells represent the effector components of the specific immune response. Antibodies are the most important protective mechanism against bacteria and they also play a role in the protection against viral infections. In particular, neutralizing antibodies play a fundamental role in preventing the infection of new cells by cell-free virus particles. However, neutralizing antibodies are not effective against cell-associated virus and, therefore, their protective role in preventing the establishment of chronic viral infections is limited. It is worthy of note that, in several virus infections where viruses are able to establish chronic infection such as cytomegalovirus (CMV) infection, the virus-specific, cell-mediated immune response is able to control the infection. Unfortunately, this is not the case for HIV-1 which is only partially controlled by the virus-specific immune response, with the exception of the long-term non-progressors (LTNP).

Interestingly, the investigation of LTNP has been instrumental for the characterization of the HIV-1-specific immune response and for the identification of the correlates of protective immunity. In this regard, we have recently shown, by the analysis of IFN-γ and IL-2 secreting cells, that three functionally distinct populations of antigen-specific CD4 T cells can be identified. This enabled us to demonstrate a skewed representation of different populations of antigen-specific CD4 T cells with a selective reduction in the proportion of HIV-1-specific IL-2 secreting CD4 T cells in HIV-1-

infected subjects with progressive as compared to non-progressive infection (Harari et al., 2004 a, b). Also of interest is that the absence of HIV-1-specific IL-2 secreting CD4 T cells was associated with that of helper cells endowed with proliferation capacity.

In addition to the functional characterization and with regard to the phenotypic characterization of memory T cells, the combined use of CCR7 and CD45RA, as shown by Sallusto et al. (1999), led to the identification of phenotypically distinct subsets of memory T cells with CCR7$^-$ T cells defining a population of effector cells (effector memory [T_{EM}]) that resides predominantly in the periphery and with CCR7$^+$ T cells (central memory [T_{CM}]) serving as precursors of effector cells and residing predominantly within the secondary lymphoid organs.

The progressive depletion of CD4 T cells is a hallmark of HIV-1 infection. In particular, the activation of effector CD4 T cells during the primary HIV-1 infection leads to their proliferation as shown by the high levels of expression of Ki67 and by the up-regulation of markers such as CCR5 (Harari et al., 2002). These two features render the effector CD4 T cells (and more importantly the HIV-1-specific CD4 T cells) more susceptible to the virus (Harari et al., 2002). In this regard, we have shown a significant difference in the magnitude of virus-specific IFN-γ secreting CD4 T cells in patients who experienced HIV-1 and CMV primary co-infection (Harari et al., 2002). The lower frequency of HIV-1-specific CD4 T cells with effector function, i.e., IFN-γ secreting, supported the hypothesis of the rapid elimination of HIV-1-specific CD4 T cells. Furthermore, the preferential infection of HIV-1-specific CD4 T cells by HIV-1 has been demonstrated by Douek et al. (2002) and they have shown that HIV-1-specific CD4 T cells represent between 1 and 10% of all infected CD4 T cells, while they represent less than 1% of total CD4 T cells.

We have further investigated and compared primary HIV-1 and CMV infection from functional and phenotypic standpoints. We have addressed the functional and phenotypic heterogeneity of HIV-1 and CMV-specific CD4 T cells during primary and chronic infections. We have observed that, in spite of the lower magnitude of the HIV-1-specific CD4 T cell response during primary infection, HIV-1 and CMV-specific CD4 T cell responses were qualitatively similar (Fig. 1.1). Both HIV-1 and CMV-specific CD4 T cell responses were mostly (> 80%) composed of single IFN-γ secreting CD4 T cells, while IL-2 secreting CD4 T cells were almost absent (Harari and Pantaleo, unpublished) (Fig. 1.1). This shows that in spite of the rapid elimination of a large number of HIV-1-specific CD4 T cells during the primary HIV-1 infection, which affects the HIV-1-specific CD4 T cells from a quantitative standpoint, the remaining HIV-1-specific CD4 T cells are comparable to CMV-specific CD4 T cells from a qualitative standpoint (Fig. 1.1). Furthermore, we have also compared HIV-1 and CMV-specific CD4 T cells during primary HIV-1 and CMV infection from a phenotypic standpoint. For these purposes, we have analyzed the distribution of HIV-1 and CMV-specific CD4 T cells within the different subsets of T cells defined by the expression of CCR7 and CD45RA. Interestingly, we have observed that both HIV-1 and CMV-specific CD4 T cells were mostly (> 90%) contained within the CD45RA$^-$CCR7$^-$ CD4 T cell population (Fig. 1.1). Therefore, overall this demonstrated that

a) in spite of their higher susceptibility to the virus and their preferential elimination, HIV-1-specific CD4 T cells can be detected during primary infection, and

b) HIV-1-specific CD4 T cells during primary HIV-1 infection are typical effector cells like CMV-specific CD4 T cells during primary CMV infection, i.e., IFN-γ secreting CD45RA$^-$CCR7$^-$ CD4 T cells.

Therefore, HIV-1 and CMV-specific CD4 T cells have the same functional and phenotypic signatures during primary infection (Fig. 1.1). We have then investigated these two functions in the context of chronic HIV-1 and CMV infections. Regarding the chronic CMV infection, we have shown that CMV-specific CD4 T cells are very heterogeneous not only from a functional but also from a phenotypic standpoint. First, we have demonstrated that, following CMV stimulation, three functionally distinct populations of antigen-specific CD4 T cells are present, i.e., single IFN-γ, IFN-γ/IL-2, and single IL-2 (Harari et al., 2004 a). Notably this functional heterogeneity was also associated with a phenotypic heterogeneity. The analysis of the distribution of CMV-specific IFN-γ and/or IL-2 secreting cells within the different subsets of CD4 T cells defined by the expression of CD45RA and CCR7 has revealed that CMV-specific cells are composed of CD45RA$^-$CCR7$^+$, CD45RA$^-$CCR7$^-$, and CD45RA$^+$CCR7$^-$ CD4 T cells (Harari et al., 2004 b; Gamadia et al., 2003) (Fig. 1.1). The IL-2 secreting cells were either CD45RA$^-$CCR7$^+$ or CD45RA$^-$CCR7$^-$ while IFN-γ secreting cells were CD45RA$^-$CCR7$^-$ and CD45RA$^+$CCR7$^-$. Therefore, chronic CMV infec-

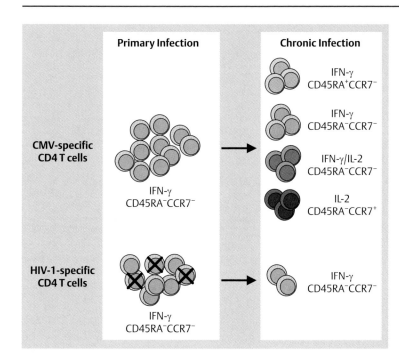

Fig. 1.1 Functional and phenotypic signatures of HIV-1 and CMV-specific CD4 T cells during primary infection.

tion is associated with a polyfunctional and multi-phenotypic CD4 T cell response (Harari et al., 2004 b) (Fig. 1.1).

HIV-1-specific CD4 T cells do not develop a similar phenotypic and functional heterogeneity as shown for CMV-specific CD4 T cells. HIV-1-specific CD4 T cells found during untreated chronic infection are functionally and phenotypically very similar to those found during primary infection, i.e., IFN-γ secreting CD45RA−CCR7− CD4 T cells (Harari and Pantaleo, unpublished) (Fig. 1.1). Therefore, chronic and progressive HIV-1 infection is associated with the same homogeneous CD4 T cell response as during primary infection (Fig. 1.1).

A recent study has suggested that to each pathogen/virus there is a corresponding type of immune response (Appay et al., 2002). We have challenged this hypothesis by analyzing the HIV-1-specific CD4 T cells response in the context of non-progressive HIV-1 infection, i.e., in LTNP. The analysis of the distribution of HIV-1-specific IFN-γ and/or IL-2 secreting cells within the different subsets of CD4 T cells defined by the expression of CD45RA and CCR7 has demonstrated that HIV-1-specific CD4 T cells in non-progressive HIV-1 infection are, like CMV-specific CD4 T cells during chronic infection, polyfunctional and multi-phenotypic. Similarly to CMV-specific CD4 T cells, the HIV-1-specific IL-2 secreting CD4 T cells in LTNP

were either CD45RA−CCR7+ or CD45RA−CCR7− while IFN-γ secreting cells were CD45RA−CCR7− and CD45RA+CCR7− (Harari et al., 2004 b).

In conclusion, HIV-1 and CMV-specific CD4 T cell responses are qualitatively similar during primary infection but very different during chronic infection. In contrast, chronic CMV and chronic non-progressive HIV-1 infections are functionally and phenotypically similar. In this regard, we have recently provided evidence that both the functional and the phenotypic heterogeneity of the antigen-specific CD4 T cells responses are influenced by antigen persistence/exposure and load (Harari et al., 2004 b; Harari et al., 2005). Therefore, the absence of qualitative differences in the HIV-1-specific CD4 T cell response between primary and chronic infection is explained by the fact that the viremia remained higher as compared to chronic CMV infection or non-progressive HIV-1 infection. The above-mentioned observations are the consequences but not the causes of the lack of control of HIV-1 viremia in progressive HIV-1 infection.

Therefore, the key question remains why is CMV replication efficiently controlled following primary infection while this is not the case in HIV-1 infection? HIV-1-specific CD4 T cells are known to play a role in the initial control of viremia following primary infection. A recent study by Gloster et al. (2004) has compared the magnitude of the HIV-1-

specific CD4 T cell response during primary HIV-1 infection with the viral setpoint in natural infection, i.e., in absence of treatment. Strong HIV-1-specific CD4 T cell responses were detected in patients who naturally established a low persisting viral load, while the responses were significantly weaker in the patients who established a high persisting viral load.

It is very likely that the initial major depletion of HIV-1-specific CD4 T cells damages the helper function to such an extent that both the humoral and the cellular (cytotoxic) immune responses are not sustained efficiently. The preferential elimination of HIV-1-specific CD4 T cells during the acute infection might also induce damages to the repertoire of the different HIV-1 epitopes recognized. In this regard, *env*-specific CD4 T cells are almost exclusively detected during early infection and are lost over time (Malhotra et al., 2003). A comprehensive analysis of the breadth of the HIV-1-specific CD4 T cell response during untreated and early primary HIV-1 infection has never been performed consistently. However, such an analysis has recently been reported by Kaufmann et al. (2004) where they have screened patients at different stages of disease with peptides spanning all HIV-1 proteins. Surprisingly, they have failed to correlate either the magnitude or the diversity, i.e., breadth, of the response with the levels of viremia.

It has been shown that early treatment of HIV-1 helps limit the massive depletion of CD4 T cells and this was associated with a more rapid recovery of HIV-1-specific CD4 T cell responses, but whether this enhances the immune control remains to be determined (Rosenberg et al., 2000). Major advances have been made in the functional characterization of HIV-1-specific CD4 T cells. However, further investigation is needed in order to identify immune correlates of protection.

References

Appay V, Dunbar PR, Callan M, Klenerman P, Gillespie GM, Papagno L, Ogg GS, King A, Lecjner F, Spina CA, Little S, Havlir DV, Richman DD, Gruener N, Pape G, Waters A, Easterbrook P, Salio M, Cerundolo V, McMichael AJ, Rowland-Jones SL. Memory CD8+ T cells vary in differentiation phenotype in different persistent virus infections. Nat Med 2002; 8: 379–385

Douek DC, Brenchley JM, Betts MR, Ambrozak DR, Hill BJ, Okamoto Y, Casazza JP, Kuruppu J, Kunstman K, Wolinsky S, Grossman Z, Dybul M, Oxenius A, Price DA, Connors M, Koup RA. HIV preferentially infects HIV-specific CD4+ T cells. Nature 2002; 417: 95–98

Gamadia LE, Remmerswaal EB, Weel JF, Bemelman F, van Lier RA, Ten Berge JJ. Primary immune responses to human CMV: a critical role for IFN-gamma-producing CD4+ T cells in protection against CMV disease. Blood 2003; 101: 2686–2692

Gloster SE, Newton P, Cornforth D, Lifson JD, Williams I, Shaw GM, Borrow P. Association of strong virus-specific CD4 T cell responses with efficient natural control of primary HIV-1 infection. AIDS 2004; 18: 749–755

Harari A, Rizzardi GP, Ellefsen K, Ciuffreda D, Champagne P, Bart PA, Kaufmann D, Telenti A, Sahli R, Tambussi G, Kaiser L, Lazzarin A, Perrin L, Pantaleo G. Analysis of HIV-1- and CMV-specific memory CD4 T-cell responses during primary and chronic infection. Blood 2002; 100 (4): 1381–1387

Harari A, Petitpierre S, Vallelian F, Pantaleo G. Skewed representation of functionally distinct populations of virus-specific CD 4 T cells in HIV-infected subjects with progressive disease: changes after antiretroviral therapy. Blood 2004a; 103: 966–972

Harari A, Vallelian F, Pantaleo G. Phenotypic heterogeneity of antigen-specific CD4 T cells under different conditions of antigen persistence and antigen load. Eur J Immunol 2004b; 34: 3525–3533

Harari A, Vallelian F, Meylan PR, Pantaleo G. Functional heterogeneity of memory CD4 T cell responses in different conditions of antigen exposure and persistence. J Immunol 2005; 174 (2): 1037–1045

Kahn JO, Walker BD. Acute human immunodeficiency virus type 1 infection. N Engl J Med 1998; 339: 33–39

Kaufmann DE, Bailey PM, Sidney J, Wagner B, Norris PJ, Johnston MN, Cosimi LA, Addo MM, Lichterfeld M, Altfeld M, Frahm N, Brander C, Sette A, Walker BD, Rosenberg ES. Comprehensive analysis of human immunodeficiency virus type 1-specific CD4 responses reveals marked immunodominance of *gag* and *nef* and the presence of broadly recognized peptides. J Virol 2004; 78: 4463–4477

Malhotra U, Holte S, Zhu T, Delpit E, Huntsberry C, Sette A, Shanarappa R, Maenza J, Corey L, McElrath MJ. Early induction and maintenance of env-specific T-helper cells following human immunodeficiency virus type 1 infection. J Virol 2003; 77: 2662–2674

Rosenberg ES, Altfeld M, Poon SH, Phillips MN, Wilkes BM, Eldridge RL, Robbins GK, D'Aquila RT, Goulder PJR, Walker BD. Immune control of HIV-1 after early treatment of acute infection. Nature 2000; 407: 523–526

Sallusto F, Lenig D, Forster R, Lipp M, Lanzavecchia A. Two subsets of memory T lymphocytes with distinct homing potentials and effector functions. Nature 1999; 401: 708–712

1.2 Immunodominance of HIV-1-Specific CD8+ T Cell Responses in Acute HIV-1 Infection

M. Lichterfeld, M. Altfeld

Introduction

The HIV-1 virus has infected more than 40 million individuals worldwide, and current estimates suggest that approximately 14,000 persons are infected each day (AIDS Epidemic Update, 2003). The use of highly active antiretroviral therapy (HAART) can dramatically prolong the life of individuals infected by HIV-1 (Palella et al., 1998) but early hopes for virus eradication have not been realized (Finzi et al., 1999). Treatment of HIV-1-infected patients with HAART, however, is limited by drug-related toxicities, high costs and drug resistance that can develop after prolonged periods of drug exposure. Protective and therapeutic vaccines able to induce strong and effective immune responses against the HIV-1 virus, therefore, still remain the most promising strategy to limit the devastating consequences of the HIV-1 epidemic.

Emerging data from observational and interventional studies in humans and animal models indicate that HIV-1-specific CD8+ T cells play a crucial role in the immune-mediated control of HIV-1 infection (Jin et al., 1999; McMichael and Rowland-Jones, 2001; Rosenberg et al., 2000; Schmitz et al., 1999). This antiviral activity of HIV-1-specific cytotoxic T cells is most apparent during acute HIV-1 infection, when the decline of HIV-1 viremia from excessive levels to the viral set point and the resolution of clinical symptoms of the acute retroviral syndrome coincide with the first appearance of these cells (Borrow et al., 1994; Borrow et al., 1997; Koup et al., 1994). Several studies suggest that HIV-1-specific T cell responses during the acute phase of the infection determine the subsequent level of viral replication and the speed of disease progression during chronic infection (Altfeld et al., 2001; Blattner et al., 2004). The analysis of factors influencing the evolution of HIV-1-specific CD8+ T cell responses in acute HIV-1 infection, therefore, represents a major challenge for the understanding of the immunopathogenesis of HIV-1 infection. In this review, we will focus on three factors impacting the priming and immunodominance of HIV-1-specific CD8+ T cell responses during primary HIV-1 infection:
a) the sequence of the inoculated viral strains,
b) the kinetics of viral protein expression and
c) the HLA class I background of the infected individual.

Viral Sequence Variations

A major characteristic of the HIV-1 virus is its dramatic genetic plasticity, which is largely due to a high error rate of enzymes responsible for the reverse transcription of the viral genome (Gaschen et al., 2002). This leads to a tremendous genetic heterogeneity of circulating viral strains and allows the virus to rapidly adapt to selection pressure mediated by either cytotoxic CD8+ T cells, neutralizing antibodies or antiretroviral pharmaceuticals (Goulder and Walker, 1999). The first evidence for the impact of viral sequence diversity on the evolution of CD8+ T cell-mediated immune responses in primary HIV-1 infection was demonstrated in the setting of viral transmission to two genetically identical hemophiliac brothers infected by the same batches of HIV-1-contaminated Factor VIII concentrates (Goulder et al., 1997). Interestingly, in spite of the genetic homology of these individuals, the HIV-1-specific CD8+ T cell responses mounted in these patients were quite dissimilar: while one of the brothers developed dominant immune responses against the HLA-A2-restricted p17 epitope SL9 and the HLA-A3-restricted p17 epitope RK9, none of these immune reactions were observed in the other patient. This differential pattern of viral epitope recognition was not associated with altered antigen presentation, but could subsequently be linked to viral mutations that were detected in the corresponding viral CD8+ T cell epitopes of the non-responding patient, while they were absent in the responding individual. Similar observations were recently reported in the context of vertical mother-to-child transmission (Goulder et al., 2001). In HIV-1-infected mothers, it was shown that viral sequence mutations in the immunodominant HLA-B27-restricted HIV-1 Gag epitope KK10 resulted in a loss of epitope recognition by CD8[+] T cells that was associated with a breakthrough of viral replication and increased risk to transmit the mutated virus to their children during pregnancy or delivery. Importantly, babies that inherited the HLA-B27 allele from their mothers and were perinatally infected with viral species containing the KK10 sequence mutation were unable to mount the otherwise immunodominant CD8[+] T cell response against the KK10 epitope and failed to reach the same degree of spontaneous viral control that is typically observed in carriers of the HLA-B27 allele who are infected with wild-type viral strains. Instead, CD8[+] T cells in these babies targeted alternative viral regions during acute infection that typically remain subdominant when the original KK10 epitope is recognized by cytotoxic T cells.

The important impact that the genetic sequence of an inoculated virus has on the hierarchy of CD8[+] T cell responses during primary HIV-1 infection was subsequently also demonstrated in the context of sexual transmission of HIV-1 between individuals expressing the frequent HLA allele A3 (Allen et al., 2004). These individuals typically generate dominant CD8[+] T cell-mediated immune responses against the two overlapping HLA-A3-restricted Gag epitopes RK9 (RLRPGGKKK) and KK9 (KIRLRPGGK) during primary HIV-1 infection. However, when patients were infected with viral strains containing a single amino acid mutation located within the RK9 epitope and flanking the C-terminal regions of the adjacent KK9 epitope, neither of these two epitopes was targeted by CD8[+] T cells during primary infection. In addition, the intracytoplasmic expression of the variant HIV-1 p17 protein prevented recognition of both epitopes by T cell clones, supporting a role for this mutation in impacting the antigen processing of one or both epitopes. Interestingly, the *in vivo* reversion of the transmitted single amino acid mutation in one subject allowed for delayed induction of both RK9 and KK9-specific CD8[+] T cell responses and suggested a considerable viral fitness compromise of the transmitted viral species, possibly due to structural constraints on key viral functions.

Overall, these data show that the transmission of viral gene mutations both inside and adjacent to CD8[+] T cell epitopes can lead to an impairment of otherwise immunodominant immune responses in acute infection. These viral gene diversifications may become fixed and lead to a transformation of previously immunodominant epitopes into less immunogenic viral regions, but apparently can also revert to their original sequence if associated with considerable fitness costs for the viral quasispecies. The genetic plasticity of the HI virus that allows it to escape from cellular immune pressure and to revert to previous genetic sequences associated with higher replicative fitness, therefore, has significant implications for the quality and efficiency of cellular immune responses in acute infection.

Kinetics of Viral Protein Expression

In addition to the sequence of the infecting virus, the kinetics by which viral proteins are expressed, processed and presented by HLA molecules on the infected cell may be important for the hierarchy by which HIV-1-specific T cell responses develop during acute infection. Several studies indicate that the expression of viral gene products during the viral life cycle following primary HIV-1 infection occurs with different kinetics in a distinct chronological order. The early expressed HIV-1 gene products include the regulatory proteins Rev and Tat as well as Nef. The primary transcript for these proteins is completely spliced mRNA which, therefore, can be readily transported from the nucleus to the cytoplasm (Klotman et al., 1991). In contrast, the structural HIV-1 proteins Pol, Env and Gag as well as the accessory HIV-1 proteins Vpr, Vpu and Vif are encoded by unspliced or single spliced mRNA, which depends on a Rev-mediated nucleocytoplasmatic transport for protein translation in the cytoplasm to occur. These differential patterns of HIV-1 gene expression result in different kinetics of HIV-1 protein biosynthesis and might have important consequences for the temporal evolution of CD8[+] T cell responses in primary HIV-1 infection.

Based on these observations, it has been hypothesized that the early expression of Nef, Rev and Tat during the viral replication cycle results in an accelerated presentation of viral epitopes within these proteins to the immune system and might thus lead to a preferential targeting of these proteins by CD8[+] T cells during acute HIV-1 infection. For instance, in a recent study from our laboratory (Lichterfeld et al., 2004a) (Fig. 1.2), a comprehensive screening for HIV-1-specific CD8[+] T cell re-

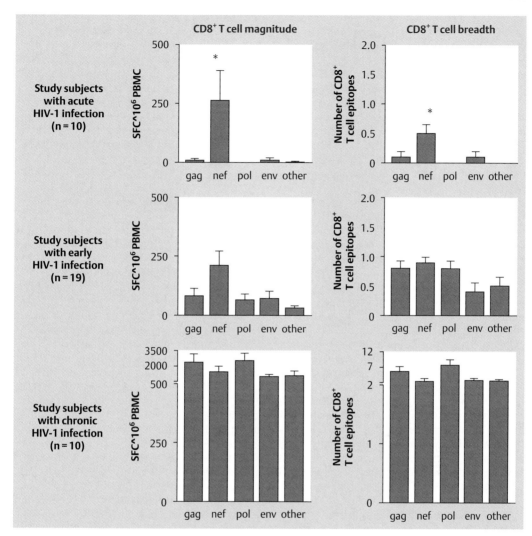

Fig. 1.2   Immunodominance of Nef-specific CD8⁺ T cell responses in primary HIV-1 infection. Diagrams summarize the magnitude and breadth of HIV-1-specific CD8⁺ T cell responses in acute HIV-1 infection, classified according to their HIV-1 protein specificity. Mean and standard deviations are shown. The early expressed protein Nef accounted for more than 90% of the total magnitude of HIV-1-specific CD8⁺ T cell responses during acute infection (Lichterfeld et al., 2004a) (* $p < 0.05$; ANOVA test of significance).

sponses with overlapping HIV-1 peptides spanning the entire HIV-1 genome revealed that Nef elicited the vast majority of CD8⁺ T cell responses during primary HIV-1 infection. Interestingly, the immunodominance of HIV-1 Nef was most prominent in individuals diagnosed early during acute HIV-1 infection prior to HIV-1 seroconversion, while a lesser degree of Nef immunodominance was seen in study persons diagnosed during primary HIV infection, thus suggesting a direct correlation be-

tween the dominance of Nef-directed CD8⁺ T cell responses and the temporal stage of primary HIV-1 infection. A high degree of Nef immunodominance was also observed in additional studies (Addo et al., 2003; Cao et al., 2003), further emphasizing the role of Nef as a preferential target of HIV-1-specific CD8⁺ T cells in acute infection. In contrast, the early expressed HIV-1 gene products Rev and Tat were only rarely described as targets for CD8⁺ T cells in acute HIV-1 infection when screening for CD8[+] T cell responses was performed using overlapping peptides derived from HIV-1-clade-specific consensus sequences or laboratory strains of HIV-1 (Addo et al., 2001; Addo et al., 2003). Given the high degree of viral diversity of Rev and Tat (Frahm et al., 2004), these findings might well refer to discrepancies between the autologous virus sequence and the viral peptide sequences that were used for CD8[+] T cell stimulation and thus did not allow one to draw definitive conclusions about the targeting of Rev and Tat by CD8[+] T cells in HIV-1 infection. Indeed, the use of overlapping HIV-1 peptides derived from the autologous viral sequence dramatically enhanced the detection of Tat-specific CD8[+] T cell responses in HIV-1 infection (Altfeld et al., 2003 b) and thus suggests that Tat might also represent a prominent target for HIV-1-specific CD8[+] T cells during the early phase of the disease.

Indirect evidence for an accelerated recognition of the early expressed HIV-1 gene products during primary HIV-1 infection has recently been provided in a series of *in vitro* experiments (Ali et al., 2004; van Baalen et al., 2002 a). In these studies, it was shown that the translocation of reverse transcriptase (RT) or Gag CD8[+] T cell epitopes into the early expressed Nef protein could dramatically enhance the ability of Gag or RT-specific CD8[+] T cell clones to suppress viral replication following primary *ex vivo* infection of isolated CD4[+] T cells. Further analysis indicated that this effect was partially attributable to the abrogation of Nef-mediated MHC class I down-regulation, but was also related to the altered timing of the presentation of the corresponding RT and Gag epitopes. Thus, the kinetics of HIV-1 protein expression can apparently fundamentally impact the time course of HIV-1 antigen recognition by HIV-1-specific CD8[+] T cells and thereby contribute to the evolution of immunodominant cellular immune responses during acute HIV-1 infection.

A prominent role for the early expressed HIV-1 proteins Tat and Nef as targets for CD8[+] T cells was also indicated during primary SIV infection in rhesus macaques. Interestingly, it was shown in two studies (Allen et al., 2000; O'Connor et al., 2003) that Nef and Tat not only elicited a significant proportion of the total magnitude of SIV-specific CD8[+] T cells, but CD8[+] T cell epitopes within these early expressed SIV gene products were also the first ones to exhibit CD8[+] T cell-induced sequence variations. Thus, CD8[+] T cells directed against Tat and Nef apparently exert strong immune pressure against the virus during primary infection. This ob-

servation might correspond to the fact that, due to early expression of their target proteins, these cells have a kinetic advantage in recognizing HIV-1-infected cells before new viral progeny has been released (Gruters et al., 2002; van Baalen et al., 2002 b). Overall, the present data suggest that the expression kinetics of HIV-1 proteins can shape the cluster of immune responses emerging during primary HIV-1 infection and therefore might be of specific interest for the rational design of HIV-1-specific vaccines.

Genetic HLA Class I Background

In addition to the timing of the expression of HIV-1 proteins during the viral life cycle, the kinetics by which these proteins are processed and epitopes are loaded and presented by HLA molecules may be crucial for the determination of immunodominance. Data from several independent cohort studies have revealed an important impact of certain HLA class I alleles on the disease progression in HIV-1-infected individuals (Carrington and O'Brien, 2003). These observations include a delay in progression to AIDS associated with HLA-B27 and HLA-B57 (Hendel et al., 1999; Kaslow et al., 1996) and an acceleration of HIV-1 disease progression conferred by HLA-B35 (Gao et al., 2001; Itescu et al., 1992). The functional basis for these genetic effects currently still remains unknown. However, recent studies suggested that HLA class I alleles with protective effects on HIV disease progression apparently have a profound impact on the evolution of dominant immune responses during acute HIV-1 infection. For instance, recent data (Altfeld et al., 2003 a) showed that the HLA-B57 allele has a dominant effect on the emergence of HIV-1-specific CD8[+] T cell responses in acute infection and might in this way significantly influence the clinical severity of the acute retroviral syndrome associated with primary HIV-1 infection. Indeed, during acute HIV-1 infection of HLA-B57-expressing individuals, CD8[+] T cell epitopes restricted by B57 were by far the most frequently targeted viral regions and significantly exceeded the number of targeted CD8[+] T cell epitopes restricted by all other HLA class I alleles together in any given individual (Fig. 1.**3**). Moreover, CD8[+] T cells directed against B57-restricted epitopes contributed consistently more than 70% to the overall magnitude of HIV-1-specific CD8[+] T cells during acute HIV-1 infection. Interestingly, this immunodominance of B57-restricted immune responses was linked to a

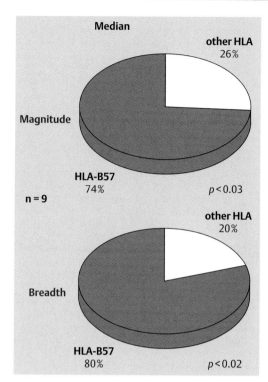

Fig. 1.**3** Contribution of HLA-B57-restricted HIV-1-specific CD8⁺ T cell responses to the total HIV-1-specific CD8⁺ T cell responses. The median contribution of HLA-B57-restricted responses to the total HIV-1-specific CD8⁺ T cell responses as well as the median contribution of responses restricted by all other HLA class I alleles is shown for magnitude *(upper panel)* and breadth *(lower panel)*. Statistical significance of differences in the magnitude and breadth between HLA-B57-restricted responses and responses restricted by all other expressed HLA class I alleles was calculated using a two-tailed *t*-test (Altfeld et al., 2003 b).

beneficial clinical presentation during acute HIV-1 infection, a low level of set point viremia and a favorable long-term disease progression. These observations have led to the hypothesis that HLA-B57 molecules might have an accelerated capacity to present HIV-1 antigens on the cell surface, which might give CD8⁺ T cells targeting HLA-B57-restricted epitopes a kinetic advantage over immune responses that subsequently evolve.

A profound impact of HLA class I alleles on CD8⁺ T cell epitope selection in acute HIV infection was also documented in others studies (Goulder et al., 1997; Yu et al., 2002). For instance, recent data from Yu et al. (2002) indicated a consistent pattern of immunodominant HIV-1-specific CD8⁺ T cell re-

sponses in individuals with an HLA-A3 or HLA-B7 background. Interestingly, these data showed that almost all (88%) carriers of HLA-A3 who mounted CD8⁺ T cell responses against HIV during primary infection targeted the HLA-A3-restricted Gag epitopes RK9 and KK9 as dominant CD8⁺ T cell epitopes, thus revealing a direct connection between the genetic HLA class I background and the hierarchy of CD8⁺ T cell responses during acute infection. A similar observation was made in carriers of HLA-B7, who consistently recognized the B7-restricted Env IL9 epitope as the immunodominant CD8⁺ T cell target during acute HIV infection (Yu et al., 2002). Importantly, the initial pattern of immunodominance both in individuals with HLA-A3 and HLA-B7 background persisted during the ensuing disease process, regardless of whether these patients were continuously treated with highly active antiretroviral therapy or were sequentially exposed to their autologous virus in structured treatment interruptions.

Finally, important evidence for the relevance of HLA class I alleles on the evolution of an immunodominant HIV-1-specific immune response in acute infection has been generated in an animal model of SIV-infected rhesus macaques (O'Connor et al., 2003). Here, it was shown that the two MHC class I alleles which are most strongly associated with a beneficial long-term SIV disease outcome in primates (Mamu A01 and Mamu B17) restricted the viral epitopes of the dominant CD8⁺ T cell responses during acute infection in animals expressing these alleles. These immune responses rapidly selected for viral escape mutations in the corresponding viral epitopes during acute infection, reflecting the strong immune pressure mediated by these cells. Overall, these data suggest that HLA class I alleles associated with slow advance to AIDS bind epitopes that are preferentially recognized in acute infection and by this mechanism might at least partially exert protective effects against HIV disease progression.

Conclusion

Recent studies indicate that both viral and host factors significantly determine the evolution of immunodominant CD8⁺ T cell responses in acute HIV-1 infection. However, these investigations have mainly identified HIV-1-specific T cell responses by means of interferon-γ secretion or staining with MHC class I tetramer complexes, which might not be directly predictive of the cytotoxic effects of these cells. Indeed, recent studies showed that the hierarchy of HIV-1-specific CD8⁺ T cell responses varies in terms of what kind of effector function of CD8⁺ T cells is analyzed (Lichterfeld et al., 2004 b), implicating that dominant interferon-γ secreting CD8⁺ T cells might only be subdominant with regard to their cytotoxic activity. The future analysis of immunodominant HIV-1-specific CD8⁺ T cell responses will therefore rely on a more comprehensive functional assessment of these cells, which will contribute to a more profound understanding of mechanisms responsible for the evolution of dominant CD8⁺ T cell responses that are associated with partial control of HIV-1 replication in acute infection.

References

Addo MM, Altfeld M, Rosenberg ES et al. The HIV-1 regulatory proteins Tat and Rev are frequently targeted by cytotoxic T lymphocytes derived from HIV-1-infected individuals. Proc Natl Acad Sci USA 2001; 98: 1781–1786

Addo MM, Yu XG, Rathod A et al. Comprehensive epitope analysis of human immunodeficiency virus type 1 (HIV-1)-specific T-cell responses directed against the entire expressed HIV-1 genome demonstrate broadly directed responses, but no correlation to viral load. J Virol 2003; 77: 2081–2092

AIDS Epidemic Update 2003, http://www.unaids.org

Ali A, Lubong R, Ng H, Brooks DG, Zack JA, Yang OO. Impacts of epitope expression kinetics and class I downregulation on the antiviral activity of human immunodeficiency virus type 1-specific cytotoxic T lymphocytes. J Virol 2004; 78: 561–567

Allen TM, O'Connor DH, Jing P et al. Tat-specific cytotoxic T lymphocytes select for SIV escape variants during resolution of primary viraemia. Nature 2000; 407: 386–390

Allen TM, Altfeld M, Yu XG, O'Sullivan KM, Lichterfeld M, Le Gall S, John M, Mothe BR, Lee, PK, Kalife, ET, Cohen DE, Freedberg KA, Strick DA, Johnston MN, Sette A, Rosenberg ES, Mallal SA, Goulder PJR, Brander C, Walker BD. Selection, transmission, and reversion of an antigen processing cytotoxic T-lymphocyte escape mutation in human immunodeficiency virus type 1 infection. J Virol 2004; 78: 7069–7078

Altfeld M, Rosenberg ES, Shankarappa R et al. Cellular immune responses and viral diversity in individuals treated during acute and early HIV-1 infection. J Exp Med 2001; 193: 169–180

Altfeld M, Addo MM, Rosenberg ES et al. Influence of HLA-B57 on clinical presentation and viral control during acute HIV-1 infection. Aids 2003 a; 17: 2581–2591

Altfeld M, Addo MM, Shankarappa R et al. Enhanced detection of human immunodeficiency virus type 1-specific T-cell responses to highly variable regions by using peptides based on autologous virus sequences. J Virol 2003 b; 77: 7330–7340

Blattner WA, Ann Oursler K, Cleghorn F et al. Rapid clearance of virus after acute HIV-1 infection: correlates of risk of AIDS. J Infect Dis 2004; 189: 1793–1801

Borrow P, Lewicki H, Hahn BH, Shaw GM, Oldstone MB. Virus-specific CD8⁺ cytotoxic T-lymphocyte activity associated with control of viremia in primary human immunodeficiency virus type 1 infection. J Virol 1994; 68: 6103–6110

Borrow P, Lewicki H, Wei X et al. Antiviral pressure exerted by HIV-1-specific cytotoxic T lymphocytes (CTLs) during primary infection demonstrated by rapid selection of CTL escape virus. Nat Med 1997; 3: 205–211

Cao J, McNevin J, Holte S, Fink L, Corey L, McElrath MJ. Comprehensive analysis of human immunodeficiency virus type 1 (HIV-1)-specific gamma interferon-secreting CD8⁺ T cells in primary HIV-1 infection. J Virol 2003; 77: 6867–6878

Carrington M, O'Brien SJ. The influence of HLA genotype on AIDS. Annu Rev Med 2003; 54: 535–551

Finzi D, Blankson J, Siliciano JD et al. Latent infection of CD4⁺ T cells provides a mechanism for lifelong persistence of HIV-1, even in patients on effective combination therapy. Nat Med 1999; 5: 512–517

Frahm N, Korber BT, Adams CM et al. Consistent cytotoxic-T-lymphocyte targeting of immunodominant regions in human immunodeficiency virus across multiple ethnicities. J Virol 2004; 78: 2187–2200

Gao X, Nelson GW, Karacki P et al. Effect of a single amino acid change in MHC class I molecules on the rate of progression to AIDS. N Engl J Med 2001; 344: 1668–1675

Gaschen B, Taylor J, Yusim K et al. Diversity considerations in HIV-1 vaccine selection. Science 2002; 296: 2354–2360

Goulder PJ, Walker BD. The great escape – AIDS viruses and immune control. Nat Med 1999; 5: 1233–1235

Goulder PJ, Sewell AK, Lalloo DG et al. Patterns of immunodominance in HIV-1-specific cytotoxic T lymphocyte responses in two human histocompatibility leukocyte antigens (HLA)-identical siblings with HLA-A*0201 are influenced by epitope mutation. J Exp Med 1997; 185: 1423–1433

Goulder PJ, Brander C, Tang Y et al. Evolution and transmission of stable CTL escape mutations in HIV infection. Nature 2001; 412: 334–338

Gruters RA, van Baalen CA, Osterhaus AD. The advantage of early recognition of HIV-infected cells by cytotoxic T-lymphocytes. Vaccine 2002; 20: 2011–2015

Hendel H, Caillat-Zucman S, Lebuanec H et al. New class I and II HLA alleles strongly associated with opposite patterns of progression to AIDS. J Immunol 1999; 162: 6942–6946

Itescu S, Mathur-Wagh U, Skovron ML et al. HLA-B35 is associated with accelerated progression to AIDS. J Acquir Immune Defic Syndr 1992; 5: 37–45

Jin X, Bauer DE, Tuttleton SE et al. Dramatic rise in plasma viremia after CD8(+) T cell depletion in simian immunodeficiency virus-infected macaques. J Exp Med 1999; 189: 991–998

Kaslow RA, Carrington M, Apple R et al. Influence of combinations of human major histocompatibility complex genes on the course of HIV-1 infection. Nat Med 1996; 2: 405–411

Klotman ME, Kim S, Buchbinder A, DeRossi A, Baltimore D, Wong-Staal F. Kinetics of expression of multiply spliced RNA in early human immunodeficiency virus type 1 infection of lymphocytes and monocytes. Proc Natl Acad Sci USA 1991; 88: 5011–5015

Koup RA, Safrit JT, Cao Y et al. Temporal association of cellular immune responses with the initial control of viremia in primary human immunodeficiency virus type 1 syndrome. J Virol 1994; 68: 4650–4655

Lichterfeld M, Yu X, Cohen D, Addo MM, Malenfant JPB, Pae E, Johnston MN, Strick DAT, Rosenberg ES, Korber BWB, Altfeld M. HIV-1 Nef is preferentially recognized by CD8+ T cells in primary HIV-1 infection despite a relatively high degree of genetic diversity. AIDS 2004a; 18: 1383–1392

Lichterfeld M, Yu XG, Waring MT et al. HIV-1-specific cytotoxicity is preferentially mediated by a subset of CD8+ T cells producing both interferon-γ and tumor-necrosis factor-α. Blood 2004b; 104: 487–494

McMichael AJ, Rowland-Jones SL. Cellular immune responses to HIV. Nature 2001; 410: 980–987

O'Connor DH, Mothe BR, Weinfurter JT et al. Major histocompatibility complex class I alleles associated with slow simian immunodeficiency virus disease progression bind epitopes recognized by dominant acute-phase cytotoxic-T-lymphocyte responses. J Virol 2003; 77: 9029–9040

Palella FJ, Jr., Delaney KM, Moorman AC et al. Declining morbidity and mortality among patients with advanced human immunodeficiency virus infection. HIV Outpatient Study Investigators. N Engl J Med 1998; 338: 853–860

Rosenberg ES, Altfeld M, Poon SH et al. Immune control of HIV-1 after early treatment of acute infection. Nature 2000; 407: 523–526

Schmitz JE, Kuroda MJ, Santra S et al. Control of viremia in simian immunodeficiency virus infection by CD8+ lymphocytes. Science 1999; 283: 857–860

van Baalen CA, Guillon C, van Baalen M et al. Impact of antigen expression kinetics on the effectiveness of HIV-specific cytotoxic T lymphocytes. Eur J Immunol 2002a; 32: 2644–2652

van Baalen CA, Stittelaar KJ, Osterhaus AD, Guillon C, Gruters RA. The choice of antigen for therapeutic immunization against AIDS. Trends Immunol 2002b; 23: 478–479

Yu XG, Addo MM, Rosenberg ES et al. Consistent patterns in the development and immunodominance of human immunodeficiency virus type 1 (HIV-1)-specific CD8+ T-cell responses following acute HIV-1 infection. J Virol 2002; 76: 8690–8701

1.3 Impact of Viral Sequence Evolution on Immune Control of HIV-1

J. Timm, T. M. Allen

Introduction

The enormous global sequence diversity of HIV-1 clearly represents one of the key hurdles in the design of an effective vaccine. This same sequence diversity presents a unique problem to the immune system by forcing it to continuously adapt to ever-changing viral quasi-species. Alignment of Gag-protein sequences of HIV-1 from the Los Alamos HIV database (http://www.hiv.lanl.gov/) to a consensus sequence illustrates this enormous diversity (Fig. 1.4). Understanding the mechanisms driving the evolution of HIV-1, and its impact on immune control and disease progression, will be important for designing effective vaccines hoping to prevent or control HIV-1 infection.

One of the components which distinguishes retroviruses such as HIV-1 from most other pathogens is their conversion of a viral RNA genome into a double-stranded DNA molecule. This process is mediated by the viral reverse transcriptase (RT), a notoriously error-prone enzyme that results in the daily production of a wide range of viral variants referred to as quasi-species. Mathematical modeling of HIV-1 replication dynamics suggests that each day virtually every possible viral variant is generated within a host (Coffin, 1995). While many of these mutations are lethal to the virus, a small proportion of changes can be beneficial, often in terms of increasing the replicative capacity of the virus or aiding its evasion of host immune responses. Viruses harboring such beneficial mutations will possess a selective advantage over others and will come to represent the dominant form of the virus in a host. This process is ongoing over the course of infection and ultimately shapes the sequence composition of the virus. While numerous studies have documented the ability of viral mutations to compromise host immune responses, the extent and impact of these escape mutations on disease progression is less well understood. Therefore, there is a need for additional studies to determine how sequence diversity of HIV-1 results in viral escape from both cellular and humoral immune responses, how transmission of these mutations affects the ability to mount immune responses during acute infection, and how sequence diversity contributes to HIV-1 superinfection and prohibits sufficient cross-reactivity of vaccine-elicited immune responses. Fortunately, with enormous advances in sequencing technologies combined with improved cellular and humoral assays to measure and characterize immune responses, we now possess more powerful tools to dissect out these intricate host-pathogen interactions.

Immune Evasion – Escaping Antibodies and T Cell Responses

Humoral and cellular immune responses together form the two arms of the adaptive host immune response designed to protect the host from invading pathogens. Neutralizing antibodies bind in a highly specific manner to small regions on the surface of a pathogen and are designed to eliminate cell-free viruses from the host. Although neutralizing antibodies can be protective in many viral infections, and form the basis for the majority of protective vaccines designed to date, this is clearly not the case in HIV-1 infection. Neutralizing antibodies appear to contribute to the control of HIV-1 over the course of infection, however they do not appear to play a role in the immediate containment of the virus (Schmitz et al., 2003). In turn, CD8[+] T cells represent one subset of the cellular adaptive immune response. CD8[+] cytotoxic T cells (CTL) function to eliminate virally infected cells, recognizing them through the interaction of specific receptors (major histocompatibility complex [MHC or HLA] and the T-cell receptor [TCR]) on the surface of both cells. The importance of the cellular immune response in the control of HIV-1 has perhaps been best illustrated in the rhesus macaque

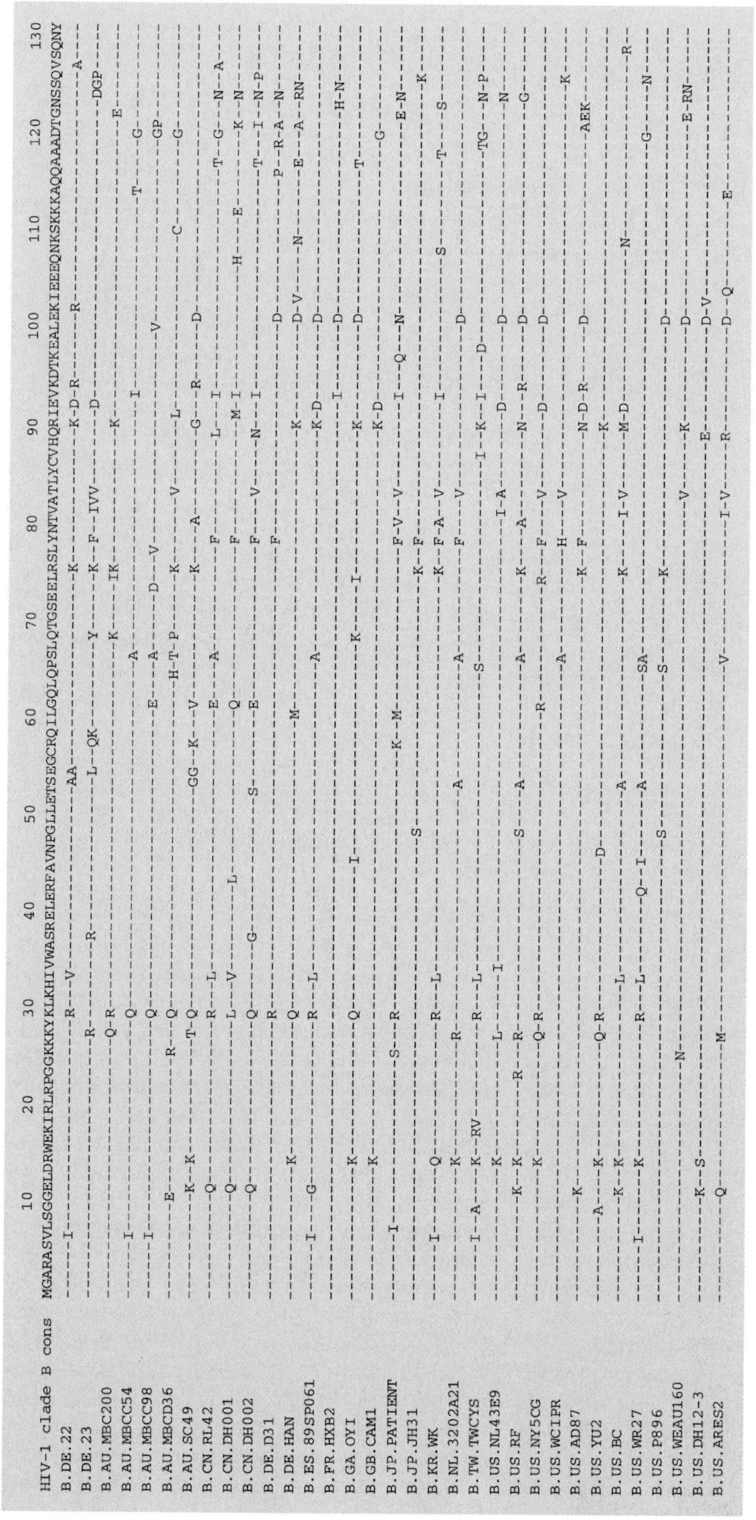

Fig. 1.4 First 132 amino acids of HIV-1 Gag-protein sequences from the Los Alamos HIV database (http://www.hiv.lanl.gov/) aligned to the HIV-1 clade B consensus sequence.

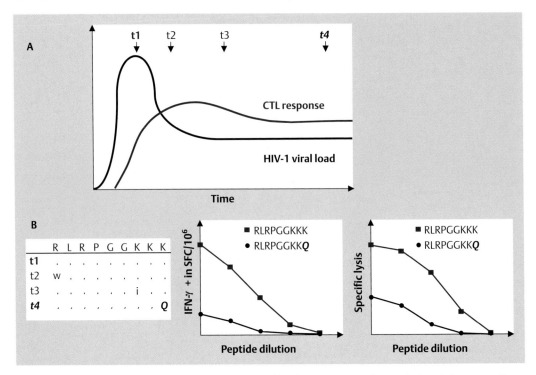

Fig. 1.**5** **a** During acute HIV-1 infection a decline in viral load to a set point after peak viremia is temporally associated with emergence of HIV-1-specific CTL responses. **b** Longitudinal sequence analysis (time points t1 through t4) of an HLA-A3 restricted CTL epitope over the course of infection reveals mutations in the targeted epitope (Allen et al., 2004 a,b). The variant with the fixed mutation in position 9 of the epitope (RLRPGGKK**Q**) displays a compromised ability to stimulate IFN-γ secretion or induce cytotoxicity compared to the early autologous epitope sequence (RLRPGGKKK).

model, where depletion of CD8[+] T cells resulted in substantial increases in viral loads of SIV-infected macaques and in faster disease progression (Matano et al., 1998; Schmitz et al., 1999; Yin et al., 1999). Moreover, the emergence of CTL responses is associated with a decline in viral load after peak viremia in the acute phase of HIV-1 infection (Fig. 1.5 a).

While the development of neutralizing antibodies is not protective, antibodies may still be contributing to the control of infection. Sequence analysis of HIV-1 reveals an enormously high variability in the surface exposed region of the envelope protein, suggestive of immune selective pressures on that region of the virus typically exposed to antibodies (Burns and Desrosiers, 1994). The first direct evidence was obtained from *in vitro* studies of HIV-1 evolution in the presence of neutralizing antibodies. Sequence analyses of the envelope region revealed mutations in antibody-targeted regions resulting in abrogated binding consistent with viral escape (Reitz et al., 1988). The relevance of antibody escape mutations has also been shown *in vivo* in humans (Albert et al., 1990) and more systematically in the rhesus macaque model (Burns et al., 1993; Choi et al., 1994; Hofmann-Lehmann et al., 2002), but efforts have been hampered by lack of techniques that allow testing of the antibody response against autologous virus. More recent approaches using pseudovirions revealed potent neutralizing antibody responses after acute infection with the development of new antibody responses arising over the course of infection in response to continuous evolution of HIV-1 (Richman et al., 2003; Wei et al., 2003). Why this selective pressure is not sufficient to contain infection in many cases is unclear, but suggests that HIV-1 is always one step ahead of the immune response.

Unlike neutralizing antibodies, which are all directed against surface-exposed regions of the viral envelope, the cellular immune responses can be directed against all proteins of the virus. Numerous HIV-1-specific CD8[+] and CD4[+] T cell epitopes, or short 8–11 amino acid stretches of a protein, have now been more extensively defined (Addo et al., 2003; Brander and Goulder, 2000; Kaufmann et al., 2004), along with the HLA alleles which specifically bind these epitopes. Most subjects appear to target dozens of different regions of HIV-1 with different CD8 and CD4 immune responses, implying an enormous effort by the immune system to control HIV-1. Similarly, numerous studies have identified the development of escape mutations in CD8 epitopes in both the SIV-infected rhesus macaque (Allen et al., 2000; Barouch et al., 2002; Evans et al., 1999; Mortara et al., 1998) but also in humans (Borrow et al., 1997; Goulder et al., 1997; Goulder et al., 2001; Phillips et al., 1991; Price et al., 1997). Even minor mutations in HIV-1 are capable of abrogating CD8 T cell responses by interfering with binding of the epitope to the HLA class I molecule on the surface of an infected cell, or by impairing the ability of the T cell receptor on the surface of CD8 T cells to recognize the altered epitope. In most studies, the impact of mutations within an epitope on T cell recognition is determined in assays that test effector functions (cytotoxicity or cytokine secretion) using dilutions of the original and variant epitopes (Fig. 1.**5b**). CTL escape mutations can be selected during both the acute (Borrow et al., 1997) and chronic phases (Goulder et al., 2001; Moore et al., 2002) of infection, suggesting that as with neutralizing antibody responses the virus is continuously evolving to evade these responses. As most studies have focused on evolution within frequently targeted or immunodominant epitopes, there still remains little data on the extent to which HIV-1 escapes from host immune responses and to what degree this impairs overall immune control of the virus. More recent approaches utilizing longitudinal full-length sequencing of HIV-1 and SIV suggest that a significant degree of mutations developing outside the envelope region of these viruses is associated with CD8[+] T cell pressures (Allen et al., 2004b; Liu et al., 2004). However, while significant work has been done to document viral escape from CD8 T cell responses in HIV-1 and SIV, we continue to lack some fundamental understanding of the degree to which viral escape is impairing overall immune control of the AIDS virus.

Impact of HIV-1 Sequence Evolution on Disease Progression

Despite numerous studies illustrating viral escape from both cellular and humoral immune responses over the course of infection, the impact that these escape mutations are having on disease progression is less well understood. The best evidence that viral escape may profoundly alter disease progression comes from studies conducted in the SHIV-infected rhesus macaque model (Barouch et al., 2002). Animals vaccinated with a candidate AIDS vaccine were able to control viral replication and prevent disease progression after challenge with a pathogenic simian-human immune deficiency virus (SHIV-89.6P). In this study the development of escape mutations within a single immunodominant CTL epitope in Gag was associated with loss of viral containment and clinical disease progression. While the study concluded that loss of viral control in these animals was associated with viral escape from this immunodominant CD8 response it is important to also consider that evolution at other sites in the virus may have also contributed to this phenomenon.

Similarly, a recent case report describes an HIV-1-infected child having mounted an immunodominant HLA-B27-restricted Gag CTL response and controlling viral replication for almost eight years (Feeney et al., 2004). Sequence analysis prior to and immediately following loss of control revealed development of a mutation in this B27-restricted CD8 epitope that was underway before viral load increased. This mutated virus was the dominant quasi-species after loss of control, coinciding with loss of the specific CD8 response. The temporal association in this case similarly suggests viral escape from a CD8 response as the cause for failure of viral containment. An association between viral escape from the same HLA-B27-restricted Gag epitope and faster disease progression to AIDS has also been previously reported (Goulder et al., 1997). However, in this latter study limited sample availability made the precise timing of CTL escape relative to loss of viral control difficult to determine. Therefore, additional studies are required to understand the true impact that particular CD8 escape mutations can have on immune control. As the CD8 epitopes targeted in each of these studies lie within uniquely conserved regions of HIV-1 and SIV, these studies begin to suggest that some particular CD8 T cell responses targeting structurally constrained regions of the virus may be uniquely able to control the AIDS virus.

Antigen Processing Mutations – An Alternative Mechanism of Immune Evasion

CD8 T cell recognition of a viral peptide or epitope is affected by the strength of the binding between the viral peptide and the HLA class I molecule (affinity) and by the T cell receptor's ability to bind to this complex (avidity). Mutations at residues of an epitope that determine HLA-binding, namely the anchor residues which typically lie at positions 2 and 9 of an epitope, impair the binding of the peptide to the HLA molecule, while mutations at the remaining residues of the peptide often impair recognition by the T cell receptor. However, both of these described mechanisms of viral escape select for mutations inside the epitope.

Alternatively, a potentially more efficient mechanism to evade the host immune system is to prevent an epitope normally recognized by the immune response from being properly generated and ever reaching the surface of the cell. Several steps are necessary before an antigenic peptide can be presented on the cell surface in complex with an HLA class I molecule. Generally this first involves degradation of the viral protein by cytosolic proteases in the proteasome (Rock et al., 1994) whose products are then further trimmed by peptidase enzymes (Saric et al., 2001; York et al., 2003). The smaller peptides are then transported into the endoplasmatic reticulum (ER) where they are loaded on the HLA class I molecule and transported to the cell surface (Lauvau et al., 1999). Several specific proteases and peptidases as well as ligand-specific transporters are also known to be involved (Neefjes et al., 1995; Saric et al., 2002; Seifert et al., 2003; Serwold et al., 2002). Recent studies on HIV-1 now directly illustrate that mutations lying outside of an epitope can alter this normal antigen processing. One study highlighted the impact of a mutation in the NH_2-terminal flanking region of the HLA-B57 restricted IW9 CTL epitope which inhibited the ability of the ER-resident aminopeptidase I (ERAP I) to trim the antigen to the correct peptide length required for binding to the HLA class I molecule (Draenert et al., 2004). The other study demonstrated a processing mutation in the C-terminal flanking region of the HLA-A3 restricted Gag epitope KK9 (Allen et al., 2004a, b). This mutation was associated with the decline of the CTL response *in vivo*, but moreover frequent transmission of this mutation to subjects expressing HLA-A3 was found to prevent the ability of these subjects to mount this normally immunodominant CD8 response, thus compromising initial responses against the virus. Therefore, these studies indicate that not only do mutations within targeted epitopes affect the ability of the immune system to recognize HIV-1, but that mutations developing elsewhere in the viral protein can have similar effects. Given that many CD8 epitopes cluster in often conserved regions of HIV-1, such antigen processing mutations may present a unique advantage to the virus through potentially silencing whole antigenic regions containing several epitopes.

Transmission and Reversion of Escape Mutations

The fate of CD8 escape mutations on a population level has important implications for the development of a vaccine. If escape mutations can be transmitted, and are stable after their transmission to a new host, then epitopes restricted by frequent HLA alleles may be deleted from viruses circulating in a population. For example, mutations known to be associated with a particular HLA molecule such as HLA-B7 can be found in an elevated frequency in patients expressing this allele compared to the general population (Moore et al., 2002). This suggests that HIV-1 is adapting to evade certain host immune responses, and that some of these mutations may be accumulating in circulating strains of HIV-1 after passage through HLA-B7-positive subjects. Because some CD8 escape mutations are being transmitted, and are expected to arise more frequently for common HLA alleles such as A2, A3, B7, one might expect that the continued passage of a virus through a population results in a more rapid accumulation of mutations associated with these frequent alleles than mutations associated with rare alleles. Indeed, one study suggests that this may be the case since individuals expressing rare HLA alleles, to which HIV-1 may be less well adapted, appear to have an advantage to control HIV-1 (Trachtenberg et al., 2003). Such issues are complicating the selection of vaccines since the impact of many of the observed sequence polymorphisms in any given strain on immune recognition of HIV-1 is largely unknown. A few mutations can be clearly attributed to specific HLA alleles and CTL responses (Allen et al., 2004a,b; Goulder et al., 2001; Moore et al. 2002), but the vast majority remain undefined.

Following cessation of antiretroviral treatment some drug resistance mutations have been shown to revert back to the original sequence (Gandhi et

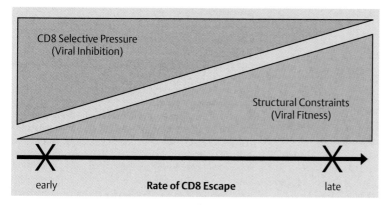

Fig. 1.**6**   The rate of evolution within a targeted epitope is largely influenced by the amount of selective pressure exerted by CD8 T cells and the degree of structural constraints in a targeted region. Strong selective immune pressure on a region with low structural constraints is expected to result in early escape mutations. A region with high structural constraints under selective immune pressure through a weak or functionally impaired CD8 response is likely to mutate more slowly.

al., 2003; Halfon et al., 2003). Two recent studies following CTL escape mutations after transmission also demonstrate the potential for reversion of mutations selected by the immune response. In one study an escape mutation residing within an HLA-B57/B5801 restricted Gag epitope was analyzed (Leslie et al., 2004). The majority of HLA-B57 or HLA-B5801-positive HIV-infected subjects eventually select for escape mutations in this epitope, but after horizontal or vertical transmission the most frequently observed mutation (T242 N) evolves back to the original sequence. However, the same study showed other mutations associated with the HLA-B57/5801 allele that did not revert back after their transmission. In the macaque model similar results have been observed (Friedrich et al., 2004). A viral clone of SIVmac239 harboring escape mutations within three immunodominant CTL epitopes was used to infect animals. Mutations that reproducibly developed later during infection reverted back to the original sequence after infection of an animal that was not able to mount the corresponding response. In contrast, a mutation in another epitope did not revert upon transmission. Therefore, as not all escape mutations seem to revert back in the absence of the force that was selecting for it, clearly other forces are at work. Overall, however, the virus harboring all three escape mutations did exhibit a reduced replicative capacity, suggesting some impact on the virus in maintaining one or more of

these mutations. Mutations impairing viral replication capacity have previously been described for drug resistance mutations (Croteau et al., 1997), suggesting that while HIV-1 may be capable of rapidly developing mutations there may be some cost associated with their development. Therefore, a state of maximal replication capacity or viral fitness is likely ultimately dependent upon the maintenance of an optimal viral protein sequence.

Escape and Fitness – the Driving Forces of Viral Evolution

CD8 escape mutations have been observed to arise with varying rates in different CTL epitopes. This likely reflects a balance between the importance of the host immune response being evaded and the impact of that mutation on the structure or function of the altered protein. As these represent competing forces acting upon the evolution of the virus, a mutation is likely to arise more rapidly if the selecting immune pressure is high and the fitness cost to the virus low. In contrast, an immune response that exerts only little selective pressure on the virus, or is directed against a region of the viral protein that is crucial for function, would take more time to drive sequence evolution (Fig. 1.**6**). Similarly, it has been described for some drug resistance and CD8 escape mutations that additional compensatory changes may develop adjacent to a mutation in order to maintain the fitness of the virus (Kelleher et al., 2001; Leslie et al., 2004; Nijhuis et al., 1999). These compensatory or neighboring mutations help to biochemically compensate the protein structure or function such that the escape mutation is better tolerated. However, as a result, escape mutations requiring compensatory mechanisms may take more time to develop. These same issues impact the degree to which certain mutations may accumulate in the population. After transmission, mutations with a relatively low fitness cost are expected to revert slowly to the original sequence or even be maintained while mutations with a high fitness cost are likely to revert more rapidly in the absence of the original selective force.

The fact that immune responses may be able to exert enough selective pressure to force the virus into a state of reduced replication capacity has important implications for the development of a vaccine. A given vaccine might not be protective as viral escape occurs, but it may contribute to viral containment and delayed disease progression by selecting for viruses with lower replication capacities. Therefore, immune responses elicited by vaccines, while primarily functioning to suppress viral replication, may provide a secondary benefit by helping to "shape" the virus into a less fit state.

Conclusions

In summary, it is clear that HIV-1 will continue to evolve on the population level as certain mutations continue to accumulate in circulating strains. Understanding which mutations are continuing to accumulate in the population, and which immune responses are impacted by these mutations, will be important to the selection of vaccine antigens. Moreover, defining the rate at which these mutations develop and/or revert may help to define particularly potent CD8 responses as well as regions of the virus which might be particularly vulnerable to immune pressures. Clearly HIV-1 possesses an enormous capacity to evolve and evade host immune responses. However, our ability to track these mutations and make light of the forces at work in shaping the evolution of HIV-1 may represent a powerful tool in helping to define limitations of this evolution.

References

Addo MM, Yu XG, Rathod A et al. Comprehensive epitope analysis of human immunodeficiency virus type 1 (HIV-1)-specific T-cell responses directed against the entire expressed HIV-1 genome demonstrate broadly directed responses, but no correlation to viral load. J Virol 2003; 77: 2081–2092

Albert J, Abrahamsson B, Nagy K et al. Rapid development of isolate-specific neutralizing antibodies after primary HIV-1 infection and consequent emergence of virus variants which resist neutralization by autologous sera. Aids 1990; 4: 107–112

Allen TM, O'Connor DH, Jing P et al. Tat-specific cytotoxic T lymphocytes select for SIV escape variants during resolution of primary viraemia. Nature 2000; 407: 386–390

Allen TM, Altfeld M, Yu XG et al. Selection, transmission, and reversion of an antigen-processing cytotoxic T-lymphocyte escape mutation in human immunodeficiency virus type 1 infection. J Virol 2004a; 78: 7069–7078

Allen TM, O'Sullivan K, Kalife ET et al. Extensive viral evolution from HIV-1 in an HLA B57+ subject and differential impact of mutations on CD8 T cell function. Whistler, Canada: Abstract, Keystone Symposium – Molecular Mechanisms of HIV Pathogenesis, 2004b

Barouch DH, Kunstman J, Kuroda MJ et al. Eventual AIDS vaccine failure in a rhesus monkey by viral escape from cytotoxic T lymphocytes. Nature 2002; 415: 335–339

Borrow P, Lewicki H, Wei X et al. Antiviral pressure exerted by HIV-1-specific cytotoxic T lymphocytes (CTLs) during primary infection demonstrated by rapid selection of CTL escape virus. Nat Med 1997; 3: 205–211

Brander C, Goulder PJ. The evolving field of HIV CTL epitope mapping: New approaches to the identification of novel epitopes. In: Korber B (ed). HIV Molecular Immunology Database 2000. Los Alamos, New Mexico: Los Alamos National Laboratory, 2000

Burns DP, Desrosiers RC. Envelope sequence variation, neutralizing antibodies, and primate lentivirus persistence. Curr Top Microbiol Immunol 1994; 188: 185–219

Burns DP, Collignon C, Desrosiers RC. Simian immunodeficiency virus mutants resistant to serum neutralization arise during persistent infection of rhesus monkeys. J Virol 1993; 67: 4104–4113

Choi WS, Collignon C, Thiriart C et al. Effects of natural sequence variation on recognition by monoclonal antibodies neutralize simian immunodeficiency virus infectivity. J Virol 1994; 68: 5395–5402

Coffin JM. HIV population dynamics in vivo: implications for genetic variation, pathogenesis, and therapy. Science 1995; 267: 483–489

Croteau G, Doyon L, Thibeault D, McKercher G, Pilote L, Lamarre D. Impaired fitness of human immunodeficiency virus type 1 variants with high-level resistance to protease inhibitors. J Virol 1997; 71: 1089–1096

Draenert R, Le Gall S, Pfafferott KJ et al. Immune selection for altered antigen processing leads to cytotoxic T lymphocyte escape in chronic HIV-1 infection. J Exp Med 2004; 199: 905–915

Evans DT, O'Connor DH, Jing P et al. Virus-specific cytotoxic T-lymphocyte responses select for amino-acid variation in simian immunodeficiency virus Env and Nef. Nat Med 1999; 5: 1270–1276

Feeney M, Tang Y, Roosevelt KA et al. Immune escape precedes breakthrough human immunodeficiency virus type 1 viremia and broadening of the cytotoxic T-lymphocyte response in an HLA-B27-positive long-term nonprogressing child. J Virol 2004; 78: 8927–8930

Friedrich TC, Dodds EJ, Yant LJ et al. Reversion of CTL escape-variant immunodeficiency viruses in vivo. Nat Med 2004; 10: 275–281

Gandhi RT, Wurcel A, Rosenberg ES et al. Progressive reversion of human immunodeficiency virus type 1 resistance mutations in vivo after transmission of a multiply drug-resistant virus. Clin Infect Dis 2003; 37: 1693–1698

Goulder PJ, Phillips RE, Colbert RA et al. Late escape from an immunodominant cytotoxic T-lymphocyte response associated with progression to AIDS. Nat Med 1997; 3: 212–217

Goulder PJ, Brander C, Tang Y et al. Evolution and transmission of stable CTL escape mutations in HIV infection. Nature 2001; 412: 334–338

Halfon P, Durant J, Clevenbergh P et al. Kinetics of disappearance of resistance mutations and reappearance of wild-type during structured treatment interruptions. AIDS 2003; 17: 1351–1361

Hofmann-Lehmann R, Vlasak J, Chenine AL et al. Molecular evolution of human immunodeficiency virus env in humans and monkeys: similar patterns occur during natural disease progression or rapid virus passage. J Virol 2002; 76: 5278–5284

Kaufmann DE, Bailey PM, Sidney J et al. Comprehensive analysis of human immunodeficiency virus type 1-specific CD4 responses reveals marked immunodominance of gag and nef and the presence of broadly recognized peptides. J Virol 2004; 78: 4463–4477

Kelleher AD, Long C, Holmes EC et al. Clustered mutations in HIV-1 gag are consistently required for escape from HLA-B27-restricted cytotoxic T lymphocyte responses. J Exp Med 2001; 193: 375–386

Lauvau G, Kakimi K, Niedermann G et al. Human transporters associated with antigen processing (TAPs) select epitope precursor peptides for processing in the endoplasmic reticulum and presentation to T cells. J Exp Med 1999; 190: 1227–1240

Leslie AJ, Pfafferott KJ, Chetty P et al. HIV evolution: CTL escape mutation and reversion after transmission. Nat Med 2004; 10: 282–289

Liu Y, Zhao H, Genowati I et al. CTL Responses as major selective forces shaping the course of HIV-1 evolution in vivo. Abstract. San Francisco: 11th Conference on Retroviruses and Opportunistic Infections, 2004

Matano T, Shibata R, Siemon C, Connors M, Lane HC, Martin MA. Administration of an anti-CD8 monoclonal antibody interferes with the clearance of chimeric simian/human immunodeficiency virus during primary infections of rhesus macaques. J Virol 1998; 72: 164–169

Moore CB, John M, James IR, Christiansen FT, Witt CS, Mallal SA. Evidence of HIV-1 adaptation to HLA-restricted immune responses at a population level. Science 2002; 296: 1439–1443

Mortara L, Letourneur F, Gras-Masse H, Venet A, Guillet JG, Bourgault-Villada I. Selection of virus variants and emergence of virus escape mutants after immunization with an epitope vaccine. J Virol 1998; 72: 1403–1410

Neefjes J, Gottfried E, Roelse J et al. Analysis of the fine specificity of rat, mouse and human TAP peptide transporters. Eur J Immunol 1995; 25: 1133–1136

Nijhuis M, Schuurman R, de Jong D et al. Increased fitness of drug resistant HIV-1 protease as a result of acquisition of compensatory mutations during suboptimal therapy. AIDS 1999; 13: 2349–2359

Phillips RE, Rowland-Jones S, Nixon DF et al. Human immunodeficiency virus genetic variation that can escape cytotoxic T cell recognition. Nature 1991; 354: 453–459

Price DA, Goulder PJ, Klenerman P et al. Positive selection of HIV-1 cytotoxic T lymphocyte escape variants during primary infection. Proc Natl Acad Sci USA 1997; 94: 1890–1895

Reitz MS, Jr., Wilson C, Naugle C, Gallo RC, Robert-Guroff M. Generation of a neutralization-resistant variant of HIV-1 is due to selection for a point mutation in the envelope gene. Cell 1988; 54: 57–63

Richman DD, Wrin T, Little SJ, Petropoulos CJ. Rapid evolution of the neutralizing antibody response to HIV type 1 infection. Proc Natl Acad Sci USA 2003; 100: 4144–4149

Rock KL, Gramm C, Rothstein L et al. Inhibitors of the proteasome block the degradation of most cell proteins and the generation of peptides presented on MHC class I molecules. Cell 1994; 78: 761–771

Saric T, Beninga J, Graef CI, Akopian TN, Rock KL, Goldberg AL. Major histocompatibility complex class I-presented antigenic peptides are degraded in cytosolic extracts primarily by thimet oligopeptidase. J Biol Chem 2001; 276: 36,474–36,481

Saric T, Chang SC, Hattori A et al. An IFN-gamma-induced aminopeptidase in the ER, ERAP1, trims precursors to MHC class I-presented peptides. Nat Immunol 2002; 3: 1169–1176

Schmitz JE, Kuroda MJ, Santra S et al. Control of viremia in simian immunodeficiency virus infection by CD8+ lymphocytes. Science 1999; 283: 857–860

Schmitz JE, Kuroda MJ, Santra S et al. Effect of humoral immune responses on controlling viremia during primary infection of rhesus monkeys with simian immunodeficiency virus. J Virol 2003; 77: 2165–2173

Seifert U, Maranon C, Shmueli A et al. An essential role for tripeptidyl peptidase in the generation of an MHC class I epitope. Nat Immunol 2003; 4: 375–379

Serwold T, Gonzalez F, Kim J, Jacob R, Shastri N. ERAAP customizes peptides for MHC class I molecules in the endoplasmic reticulum. Nature 2002; 419: 480–483

Trachtenberg E, Korber B, Sollars C et al. Advantage of rare HLA supertype in HIV disease progression. Nat Med 2003; 9: 928–935

Wei X, Decker JM, Wang S et al. Antibody neutralization and escape by HIV-1. Nature 2003; 422: 307–312

Yin C, Wu MS, Pauza CD, Salvato MS. High major histocompatibility complex-unrestricted lysis of simian immunodeficiency virus envelope-expressing cells predisposes macaques to rapid AIDS progression. J Virol 1999; 73: 3692–3701

York IA, Mo AX, Lemerise K et al. The cytosolic endopeptidase, thimet oligopeptidase, destroys antigenic peptides and limits the extent of MHC class I antigen presentation. Immunity 2003; 18: 429–440

2 New Approaches

2.1 Immune-Based Therapies in the Treatment of HIV/AIDS

L. M. Kelly, J. Lisziewicz, F. Lori

Introduction

Even though HAART (highly active antiretroviral therapy) has greatly improved the clinical outcome for HIV-1-infected patients, it is evident that it will not be able to entirely eliminate the virus from latent pools. Thus, infected individuals will likely spend decades on different HAART regimens and, unfortunately, as patient longevity increases, so do the risks of drug-related toxicity and drug failure (mutant escape). The search for alternative strategies to HAART continues and has led to some interesting studies with therapies that include *vaccine strategies* to induce cellular immunity and *immune modulators* such as virostatics or interleukins. Future therapeutic HAART regimens will likely include the addition of one or more of these or a combination may even replace HAART as maintenance therapy.

Therapeutic Vaccine Strategies

A vaccine may be defined as an immunogenic substance intended to stimulate the body's own defenses. Most "classic" *preventive* vaccines rely on the production of vaccine-generated antibodies for humoral protection against invading microorganisms. The primary HIV antigenic target has been the envelope glycoprotein gp120; antibodies that bind to this site on the virus can block viral entry. However, regardless of the different strategies utilized to raise neutralizing antibodies to this target, poor accessibility of the receptor binding site, heavy glycosylation of gp120 and viral escape due to antigenic variation have hindered the successful generation of these antibodies (Amara et al., 2002). On the other hand, *therapeutic* vaccines are designed to boost or expand an existing cellular response in patients with an established infection, in the hope that they may limit or even permanently discontinue therapy. Although individuals infected with HIV will clearly have viral proteins in their bodies, therapeutic immunization is thought to augment or provoke *de novo* responses by restoring efficient presentation of antigenic viral epitopes.

In order to mediate an effective Th-1-like cellular CTL response, antigenic epitopes must be presented to CD8[+] T cells by class I MHC molecules (Piazza et al., 2002). Therefore, for immunization purposes, these antigens must be delivered into APCs. If they are DNA encoded, they must be delivered by a viral vector or other delivery vehicle and subsequently synthesized and processed within the APC cytoplasm. Alternatively, short peptides containing T lymphocyte CTL epitopes can bind to MHC class I molecules without further cellular processing, but require delivery by a potent immunological adjuvant (Aichele et al., 1990; Fayolle et al., 1991). Besides the choice of adjuvant, viral vector or delivery vehicle, other important considerations in vaccine design include: the number of epitopes presented, route of administration (i.e., intravenous, intramuscular, intradermal needle injection, gene gun) and the feasibility of the eventual clinical application. Some vaccine strategies which have been recently evaluated for CTL responses in murine and *rhesus monkey* models include: (i) cytokine-augmented DNA vaccines; (ii) viral vectors and heterologous or homologous prime-boost strategies; (iii) lipopeptide; (iv) *ex vivo* dendritic cell (DC)-based, and (v) DC-targeted vaccines. Most of the initial studies have been carried out in the setting of preventative immunizations, however this set of data can also be used to design meaningful therapeutic vaccines.

DNA Vaccines and Cytokine Augmentation

DNA vaccines are ideal vaccines for stimulating cellular immunity, because they express antigens inside the cell, thereby presenting antigenic epitopes through a classic MHC I presentation pathway. One of the pioneering research groups in HIV DNA vaccination studies performed a dose-escalating, phase I clinical trial with an HIV-1 plasmid vaccine encoding *env* and *rev* (APL-400–003) (MacGregor et al., 2002). The vaccine was found to be well-tolerated and did not generate any significant toxicity or anti-nuclear or anti-DNA antibodies. However, CTL Th-1-like responses were observed only in the high-dose cohort. Based on this study, the authors proposed that an improved vaccine response could be possible with the use of vectors that increase protein expression and the co-administration of cytokines.

It is now generally accepted that specific cytokines may skew immunologic outcome (i.e., Th-1 or Th-2). One example is IL-2 which has been indicated as a co-stimulator of T cell effector responses and has been shown to increase vaccine-elicited responses (McAdam et al., 2000) in various murine models (Barouch et al., 2000). Accordingly, Barouch et al. compared the protective efficacy and immunogenicity of *env/gag* plasmid DNA vaccine alone to *env/gag* plasmid DNA vaccines augmented with either IL-2 immunoglobin cytokine fusion protein or IL-2 immunoglobin plasmid (Barouch et al., 2000). Seven of eight animals immunized with IL-2-augmented DNA maintained effective viral control for more than two years after challenge. The excitement over these results was, however, dampened by the report of one animal which progressed to AIDS after the emergence of a resistant strain (Barouch et al., 2002; Barouch and Letvin, 2002). A single point mutation within an immunodominant Gag CTL epitope facilitated immune escape even though the animal had an undetectable viral load (VL). Consequently, immune escape represents a major limitation for any DNA vaccine that provides CTL-specific protection based on a small number of HIV epitopes.

DNA Prime/Viral Vector Boost Strategy

Another means to improve the immunogenicity of DNA vaccines are heterologous prime-boost strategies, which combine immunization regimens. A plasmid vector is employed to transfer genetic material (prime), followed by a second presentation with a viral vector (boost). The order of presentation, DNA prime followed by viral vector boost, seems to be critical to the response. The prime-boost strategy is easily modeled in the context of preventive immunization, but may also be extended to the therapeutic setting, including the case when one considers the circulating virus as the "prime".

Modified vaccinia Ankara (MVA) vector is a highly attenuated strain of the vaccinia virus, which has lost its ability to replicate in primate cells and has proven to be a highly effective expression vector (Amara et al., 2002). Amara et al. evaluated the long-term efficacy of DNA priming and poxvirus boosting (MVA) to protect against pathogenic mucosal challenge (Amara et al., 2001; Amara and Robinson, 2002). Inoculations and boost were delivered intradermally *(i.d.)* or intramuscularly *(i.m.)* by a needle-less jet injection device. Animals were challenged seven months later with the pathogenic strain SHIV-89.6 P. It was observed that DNA immunizations raised low levels of memory cells which expanded to high frequencies within one week of the rMVA boost. The magnitude of both humoral and cellular responses was found to increase significantly with dose, while the route of administration was found to effect only humoral responses, with intradermal delivery yielding a ten-fold greater antibody response (Amara et al., 2001; Amara and Robinson, 2002). These results were more favorable than those obtained with DNA only (Egan et al., 2000) or rMVA alone (Ourmanov et al., 2000).

In another study, Shiver et al. comparatively assessed *Rhesus macaque* immune responses to HIV Gag utilizing five different vectors: three plasmid DNA vectors, modified vaccinia Ankara MVA virus vector and replication-incompetent adenovirus type 5 vector (Ad5) in a single or multiple modality (Shiver et al., 2002). Each test vector (delivered by *i.m.* injection) expressed the identical SIV_{mac239} *gag* gene which is codon optimized for expression in mammalian cells.

Animals immunized with the Ad5 vector alone, or as a booster, after priming with a DNA vector exhibited higher levels of circulating HIV-specific $CD8^+$ T cells than animals vaccinated with the other plasmid vectors. Moreover, each animal treated with a homologous or heterologous prime boost containing Ad5 has demonstrated long-term control of VL. Notably, serum samples after challenge revealed no neutralizing antibodies in all the Ad5 animals until day 42, indicating that initial viral control was cellular rather than humoral (Shiver et al., 2002). The authors concluded that early mitigation of viral infection was due solely to the vaccine elicited *gag*-specific cellular responses.

ALVAC is another virus vector which is being tested for safety and immunogenicity at multiple sites in the USA and Uganda. The canarypox virus vector efficiently infects APCs and has a self-limiting replication cycle in mammalian cells. The latter feature confers a high degree of safety to the construct (Gupta et al., 2002; Jin et al., 2002). The recombinant virus vaccine (ALVAC-HIV vCP205) expresses HIV-1 *gag, env* gp120, the transmembrane portion of gp41 and the protease coding sequence of *pol*. The randomized, double-blind, multi-center trials compared CTL responses between high and low-risk groups, sequential versus simultaneous dosing and antibody responses in vaccinia-exposed and naive patients (Gupta et al., 2002). At one site, one hundred and fifty HIV-1-seronegative subjects were randomized to eight different treatment groups with varying dose and regimen schedules. CTL responses were analyzed by chromium release assay and were found to induce a durable response which was related in magnitude to the number of doses. Neutralizing antibodies were detected in 95% of vaccinated subjects, with higher titers in vaccinia-naive groups and in patients who received a canarypox prime and gp120 boost (Gupta et al., 2002).

Even though these virus vectors exhibited a strong cellular immune response to immunization, they bear some intrinsic disadvantages: (i) pre-existing immunity to certain vectors might interfere with their immunogenicity in humans (i.e., approximately one-half of the current US population is immune to Ad5 and a large portion of the worldwide population has been vaccinated against smallpox); (ii) virus vectors have size limitations to ensure virus vector stability. This restriction in size will likewise limit the number of epitopes that may be included.

HIV Lipopeptide Vaccines

In general, lipopeptide vaccines consist of synthetic peptides containing the immunogenic epi-

tope(s) of interest, covalently linked to a fatty acid moiety(ies) (BenMohamed et al., 2002). Although the mechanism of action is as yet not well defined, Andrieu et al. have demonstrated two different cross-presentation pathways for lipopeptide uptake by DC (Andrieu et al., 2003). Peptides are first endocytosed by the antigen-presenting DC and some rely on further processing in a DC proteosome, but regardless of processing, lipopeptides are efficiently presented by class I MHC molecules to CD8$^+$ cells (Andrieu et al., 2003).

In 2001, the preliminary results from the VAC 04 ANRS phase I, randomized, open label, dose-escalating trial were published (Pialoux et al., 2001). The study was designed to test the clinical tolerance and dose regimen of the combination of six lipopeptides (Singh and O'Hagan, 1999). Twenty-eight healthy volunteers received intramuscular injections with the mixture of peptides. Proliferative responses and CD8$^+$-mediated cytotoxic activity were observed in the majority of patients.

Preliminary data have been presented by Levy et al. from another phase I clinical trial (ANRS 093) in which ALVAC was delivered in combination with Lipo-6 T (six lipopeptides containing HIV-1 epitopes from Nef, Gag and Env [Pialoux et al., 2001]). This study was designed to investigate the immunogenicity of the combination after HAART discontinuation. Seventy patients treated for at least one year with HAART alone or in combination with IL-2 were randomized to continue HAART alone or continue HAART in combination with ALVAC and Lipo-6 T. Patients received four immunizations followed by three cycles of IL-2. Patients were then offered the option of discontinuing therapy at week 40 if their VL was < 50/µl. Based on proliferative responses to p24 and time to virological failure, Levy et al. reported better control of HIV replication after cessation of therapy in the vaccinated cohort. They propose that this effect was the result of a sustained multi-epitopic HIV immune response. Although this vaccine strategy similarly demonstrated immunological control for a limited amount of time in an intent-to-treat analysis, the size and number of epitopes that may be presented also limit this vaccine vector.

Dendritic Cell-Based Immunization

In order to potentiate an HIV-specific CTL response with vaccine therapy, the importance of delivery vehicle choice and route of administration should not be overlooked. To refine cell targeting, we may take advantage of the fact that DNA vehicles and viral vectors exhibit different cell tropisms and these target cells express particular Th-1 and Th-2-like cytokines. Moreover, the level of transfection in these various cell types is not equivalent (Puaux and Michel, 2003). For example, although the adenovirus viral vector can infect a broad range of cells (Shiver et al., 2002), some cell types are resistant to this vector due to their low expression of specific adenovirus receptors (i.e., skeletal and smooth muscle, hematopoietic cells and monocyte-derived DC) (Barnett et al., 2002). By directly targeting APC, not only do the odds of correctly presenting antigen increase, but the induction of cytokines may also be more precise. Expression of vaccine DNA in non-antigen-presenting cells also limits the efficacy of the vaccine, and may increase its toxicity. The Langerhans cell layer (immature DC class) is located directly below the stratum corneum and any type of needle delivery is likely to miss this rich source of APC precursors. However, these cells may be generated from autologous PBMC, antigen loaded and re-infused into the same patient or alternatively they may be directly targeted by a simple topical delivery.

Ex Vivo Dendritic Cell-Based Immunization

Lu et al. investigated immune responses in the Chinese *Rhesus macaque* model with aldrithiol-2 (AT-2) inactivated SIV_{mac251}-pulsed DC. AT-2 modifies viral nucleocapsid proteins without disrupting the natural conformation of viral glycoproteins (Rossio et al., 1998; Lu et al., 2003). This results in an attenuated virus which is capable of binding target cells, but replication is halted before reverse transcription (Bhardwaj and Walker, 2003). Since DC are still capable of processing and presenting antigens from non-replicating virus, this has proved a useful experimental model.

Animals were intravenously inoculated with SIV_{mac251}. Fifty-six days after infection animals were subcutaneously injected with autologous DC, which had been previously isolated, cultured and pulsed with AT-2-inactivated HIV. Animals were boosted every other week for eight weeks. A decrease in VL was noted as early as ten days after the first immunization. All ten vaccinated animals displayed a significant increase in CD4+ counts, which did not seem to be related to VL. The frequency of SIV-specific memory T cells (SMTC) increased six-fold after the third immunization, then decreased and remained two-fold above

baseline values. Additionally, a significantly higher increase in cytolytic activity of SIV-specific effector T cells was observed in vaccinated animals as compared to controls. The authors propose that the first increase in circulating SMTC 10–24 days after the first immunization probably reflected stimulation of pre-existing memory T cells by the vaccine, whereas the strong responses at days 30–45 result from priming of the naive T cell pool (Lu et al., 2003). These data and conclusions support the notion that even in the presence of abundant circulating endogenous virus, the priming of naive T cells may require the authentic presentation of antigens (Lisziewicz et al., 2003).

These results are very encouraging but should be followed up to evaluate longevity of response with respect to immune escape. Another concern is the investigators' choice of animal model, which may confound the analysis of the results. The natural course of infection has not been well-characterized in Chinese macaques and the consistent VL and CD4+ results observed during the acute phase are not characteristic of SIV_{mac251} infection in macaques of Indian origin (Bhardwaj and Walker, 2003). Moreover, these animals were treated in the early stages of disease course (56 days after infection) and it has been widely demonstrated that control may be achieved with HAART or STI alone before the onset of chronic infection (Lori et al., 2000).

These results validate the usefulness of therapeutic DC immunization; however, *ex vivo* manipulation of autologous DC is a cumbersome, not yet standardized, and costly procedure which will preclude the treatment of large patient populations. Improvements in immunization delivery and choice of antigenic material may indeed improve the cellular response, as evidenced in the next section.

Direct Targeted Dendritic Cell Topical Immunization

It has been recently demonstrated that HIV-specific T cell-mediated immunity might be induced using autologous wild-type virus as a "vaccine" (autovaccination) (Lisziewicz et al., 2003). In the setting of structured treatment interruptions (STI), VL is suppressed during the "on" phase of therapy and usually rebounds during the "off" period. This intermittent, controlled exposure to HIV is thought to boost the HIV-specific immune response and is thereby referred to as "autovaccination" (Lori and

Lisziewicz, 2001). In macaques with acute SIV_{mac251} infection, STI or HAART, causing VL rebound during initial interruptions, ultimately led to complete control of viremia after permanent interruption of therapy, and was associated with the development of strong HIV-specific T cell responses (Lori et al., 2000). Similar results have been obtained in HIV-infected individuals, when treated with HAART within three months of infection (Lisziewicz et al., 1999; Rosenberg et al., 2000). However, treatment interruption did not induce immune control (auto-vaccination) in either primates or human subjects when HAART was initiated at later stages of infection (Lori and Lisziewicz, 2001). It is possible that expression of the wild-type virus by DC and activation of naive T cells, as occurs during primary infection (Rowland-Jones, 1999), is the critical element that leads to induction of protective T cell-mediated immunity.

DermaVir is a therapeutic DNA vaccine that was designed to mimic the expression of wild-type virus in DC in order to reproduce the immunological benefits of autovaccination. Based on the premise that STI viral rebound with autologous virus during the chronic phase primarily activates memory T cells, we propose that immunization with a "heterologous" HIV virus specifically targeted to DC should activate naive T cell pools (Fig. 2.1). The DermaVir vaccine, which is applied directly onto slightly exfoliated skin, is formulated with three components, plasmid DNA, encoding a full-length replication and integration-defective HIV complexed with polyethyleneimine-mannose (PEIm), a chemical polymer in a glucose solution.

Pre-clinical studies with $DermaVir_{SHIV}$ were performed in SIV-infected non-human primates. Seven *Rhesus macaques* showing signs of AIDS were randomized to receive continuous HAART or HAART STI plus three DermaVir immunizations. HAART STI did not suppress virus replication; however, when DermaVir (0.1 mg DNA) was topically administered to the four study group animals during the "on" phase of the subsequent cycles, the median rate of VL rebound sharply decreased from 0.26 to 0.09, 0.01 log/day and then to undetectable levels.

A second randomized, controlled study was performed with twenty SIV_{mac251} infected *Rhesus macaques* (Lisziewicz et al., 2005 a, b). In this study, animals were infected with SIV_{mac251} similar to the previous experiment, but treatment was started six months after infection during the chronic stage of infection. These animals were randomized to HAART STI alone or to receive $DermaVir_{SHIV}$ during

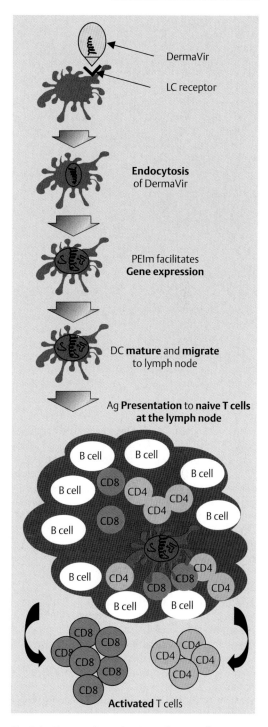

Fig. 2.1 Proposed mechanism of action for DC-targeted immunization "DermaVir"; LC = Langerhans cell; DC = dendritic cell.

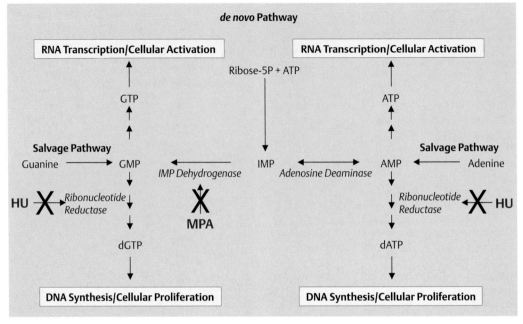

Fig. 2.**2**   General synthesis scheme for purines. Hydroxyurea (HU) inhibits ribonucleotide reductase, thus limiting the production of deoxynucleotides and blocking primarily DNA synthesis. Mycophenolic acid (MPA) targets inosinate (IMP) dehydrogenase and guanylate (GMP) production, thus effecting both RNA transcription and DNA synthesis.

the HAART phase of STI. Once again the combination of DermaVir$_{SHIV}$ and STI induced the progressive containment of VL rebound. The number of SIV-specific T cells, negligible prior to initiation of antiretroviral therapy, significantly increased during treatment and then decreased during permanent treatment interruption.

Immune Modulators

In addition to the progressive loss of CD4 T cells, a generalized qualitative impairment of lymphocyte function has been observed during HIV disease progression. Thus, in order to slow immune pathology, more consideration is now being given to the reconstitution of the immune system by increasing the number and restoring or improving biological function of T cell subsets. It is also vital that we establish new protocols for HAART which may be sustained for very long periods. These maintenance therapies should have a low toxicity profile, as well as being less prone to viral resistance. The use of immune modulators to treat HIV immune activation may allow the patient time to

recuperate naive T cell pools which are essential for survival and at the same time limit the expansion of virus and virus-targeted cells.

The first two pharmaceuticals (virostatics) described in this section chiefly exert their cytostatic effects through the inhibition of cellular enzymes involved in the formation of purines. Mycophenolic acid (MPA) and hydroxyurea inhibit purine synthesis (Fig. 2.**2**), for which there exist two pathways: de novo and salvage, and which are dependent on specific enzymes (Lori, 1999; Margolis et al., 1999). These enzymes are expressed in varying concentrations in different cell types, thus restricting pathway usage. In general, activated lymphocytes are obligated to utilize de novo pathways (resting T cells may use salvage pathways), while neurons use primarily salvage pathways and many other cell types have an equal representation of both pathway-associated enzymes (Allison and Eugui, 2000). These ribonucleotides may then i) be phosphorylated and used in transcription, or ii) be reduced by ribonucleotide reductase and subsequently phosphorylated forming the corresponding DNA deoxynucleotides (dNTP).

Since each of these drugs (MPA and hydroxyurea) reduces the synthesis of a particular nucleotide(s), the accepted rationale is to combine each of them with the nucleoside analogue which corresponds to the nucleotide eliminated from the cellular pool. Nucleoside analogues indeed inhibit the activity of HIV-1 reverse transcriptase (RT) by competing with the natural dNTP substrate for incorporation into viral DNA, and their relative concentration is increased when the natural dNTP counterpart is decreased. For example, abacavir is a carbocyclic synthetic nucleoside analogue which is converted intracellularly to its active metabolite, carbovir triphosphate, a dGTP analogue. Thus MPA, which reduces the intracellular content of dGTP, is combined with abacavir. Similarly, hydroxyurea mainly reduces the intracellular content of dATP; thus it is usually prescribed with didanosine (ddI), a precursor of the dATP analogue, dideoxyadenosine triphosphate (ddATP).

Each drug acts at a different point in the synthesis sequence; thus there are substantial differences between the various drug regimens. For instance, MPA acts early on and has an effect on both transcription and DNA synthesis, whereas hydroxyurea, which interferes with ribonucleotide reductase, primarily affects DNA synthesis (Fig. 2.**2**). Data from recent *in vitro* and *in vivo* studies clearly indicate that these drugs also effect other changes at the molecular level in various cell types. This is not surprising, since purines not only serve as precursors for DNA/RNA synthesis, but also play an important role in lipid synthesis, protein glycosylation and serve as a source of energy for many other metabolic processes. These changes may or may not be useful in the treatment of HIV.

Hydroxyurea

Hydroxyurea has been in use for more than forty years in hematology, originally for the treatment of myeloproliferative disorders, and has recently been approved for the treatment of sickle-cell anemia. Hydroxyurea utilizes multiple mechanisms of action to impede HIV replication. Firstly, hydroxyurea inhibits the cellular enzyme ribonucleotide reductase, thus blocking the transformation of ribonucleotides into deoxyribonucleotides, depleting the intracellular deoxynucleotide triphosphate (dNTP) pool, and arresting the cell cycle in the G1/S phase (Gao et al., 1993; Gao et al., 1994; Johns and Gao, 1998), thus directly halting HIV DNA synthesis. Secondly, synergistic anti-HIV activity has

been demonstrated when hydroxyurea is combined with nucleoside reverse transcriptase inhibitors (NRTI) (Lori and Lisziewicz, 1994; Malley et al., 1994; Lori et al., 1998; Palmer et al., 1999). This augmentation in antiretroviral activity may be explained by a favorable change in the proportion of activated NRTI (ddNTP) to dNTP and an enhancement of NRTI phosphorylation (Gao et al., 1995). Because NRTI compete with cellular dNTP for incorporation into the growing HIV DNA, using hydroxyurea to decrease the concentration of cellular dNTP creates a competitive advantage for the NRTI (Gao et al., 1993). Consequently, a higher proportion of the NRTI eventually becomes incorporated by reverse transcriptase into viral DNA and thus blocks DNA synthesis.

Thirdly, since cell division must progress to the G1 b phase of the cell cycle for completion of HIV reverse transcription (Korin and Zack, 1998), the virus will only replicate in activated T lymphocytes (Stevenson et al., 1990; Zack et al., 1990). Thus, when T lymphocytes are treated with hydroxyurea, they remain quiescent and become refractory to productive HIV infection. It has been proposed that the initial decrease of CD4 T lymphocytes after primary infection might account for the decrease in VL to a "set point" (Phillips, 1996). Some models also predict that the expansion of HIV is target-cell-limited (McLean et al., 1991; McLean and Nowak, 1992; Wein et al., 1998), and other models suggest that reducing target cell availability can stifle the outgrowth of drug-resistant HIV mutants (de Jong et al., 1996; De Boer et al., 1998).

Fourthly, the paradoxical restoration of immune function by the use of a cytostatic and potentially immune-suppressive drug might be explained by the following analogy. The immune system during chronic infection may be compared to an overheated automobile engine and at some point it has a higher chance of failing. This analogy is based on the realization that immune activation accompanies HIV/SIV infection and plays a fundamental role in HIV pathogenesis, possibly through multiple mechanisms, such as deleting both reactive T cells (Ameisen and Capron, 1991; Meyaard et al., 1992) and bystander cells which are not infected by the virus (Finkel et al., 1995), increasing susceptibility to apoptosis (Gougeon et al., 1996), activating "auto-immunity" (Zinkernagel and Hengartner, 1994) and reducing the generation of long-lived potential progenitor T cells (Hellerstein et al., 2003). It has also been shown that T cell activation is more closely associated with disease progression than plasma burden during HIV infection

(Giorgi et al., 1999), and CD4 T cell depletion correlates more closely with levels of immune activation than VL (Sousa et al., 2002). The immune system overactivation-pathogenesis relationship has also been confirmed in the SIV model, showing that an increased turnover in the lymph node compartments is driven by a generalized immune activation (Sopper et al., 2003).

Mycophenolic Acid

Mycophenolate mofetil (CellCept™), the pro-drug of mycophenolic acid (for simplicity we will only use the name mycophenolic acid, MPA), is licensed for the prevention of renal transplant rejection and has been extensively investigated in different models of allogeneic transplantation, autoimmune skin disorders and rheumatoid arthritis (Lui et al., 1998; Margolis et al., 1999; Colic et al., 2003). Its principal mechanism of action is the inhibition of inosine monophosphate dehydrogenase (IMPDH), which is the rate-limiting enzyme in the *de novo* synthesis of guanosine nucleotides. Additionally, it has been shown to induce apoptosis in activated T lymphocytes, suppress glycosylation and the expression of some adhesion molecules, impair differentiation and maturation of monocyte and bone-derived DC as well as inhibit primary humoral responses (Frieling and Luger, 2002).

The development of MPA as an immune-based therapy has been built upon three important observations. Firstly, it has been noted that the pool of nucleoside intermediates and deoxynucleotides allosterically regulates the key enzymes (PRPP synthetase and ribonucleotide reductase) in the production of GTP and ATP. Therefore, it may be inferred that sufficient levels of guanosine nucleotides are required for cellular proliferation (Allison and Eugui, 2000). Secondly, as previously mentioned, rapidly dividing lymphocytes depend on *de novo* dNTP synthesis, which is inhibited by MPA. Thirdly, there also exist different isoforms of IMPDH (types I and II); type I is expressed in resting lymphocytes, whereas type II is primarily expressed in activated lymphocytes and is five times more sensitive to MPA (Konno et al., 1991; Nagai et al., 1992; Allison and Eugui, 2000). Furthermore, the relative concentration of IMPDH is greater in the thymus and spleen, even with regard to tissues that are rapidly dividing, such as testis and bone marrow (Allison and Eugui, 2000). Therefore, MPA should limit cellular proliferation as well as the expansion of viruses primarily in activated T lymphocytes.

Rapamycin

Rapamycin (RAPA) is a macrocyclic triene antibiotic, which has been currently approved for the treatment of renal transplantation rejection. This immune modulating drug exerts its cytostatic effects in T cells by forming a complex with the FRAP effector, thus inhibiting IL-2 and other growth-promoting cytokines. Based on the fact that CCR5 expression is highly dependent on signaling through the IL-2 receptor, experiments have been conducted to evaluate which indirect effects RAPA may have on HIV-1 replication (Heredia et al., 2003). At concentrations as low as 1 nM, RAPA was found to reduce CCR5 surface expression on T cells, and at even lower concentrations (0.01 nM) it was sufficient to reduce CCR5 expression on monocytes. This reduced CCR5 expression correlated with a significant increase in β-chemokines, MIP-1α and MIP-1β from PBMC supernatants. Additionally, in order to assess the antiviral activity of RAPA, PBMC were cultured for seven days and then infected with either X4 or R5 strains in the presence of RAPA for an additional seven days. The authors observed a disproportionate antiviral effect in R5 virus; at 1 nM all R5 strains were inhibited by > 90% (Heredia et al., 2003). In contrast, at 10 nM RAPA, X4 strains were inhibited by 13.5%. RAPA was also found to enhance the antiviral activity of the CCR5 antagonist TAK-779.

IL-2

Although the mechanism by which IL-2 treatment increases CD4 T cells (but not CD8 cells) is not fully understood, it has been shown that this increase occurs by the peripheral expansion of existing naive CD4 T cell populations rather than by increased thymic output. Importantly, the potential for cell division in these cells is not diminished (Natarajan et al., 2002). The intermittent administration of IL-2 to patients receiving continuous HAART has also been shown to substantially decrease replication-competent HIV in resting CD4 T cells (Chun et al., 1999). Silvestri and coworkers (Paiardini et al., 2001) demonstrated that the exogenous administration of IL-2 to lymphocytes "restores the phase-specific pattern of expression of cell cycle-dependent proteins and is associated with low levels of apoptosis". In particular, while normal rates of IL-2 production are observed during HIV infection, its functionality is impaired 2- to 3fold, but the addition of IL-2 normalizes this defective biological activity (Paiardini et al., 2001). This drug should, however, be used with caution in patients with advanced disease since NIAID studies indicate that IL-2 can accelerate disease progression in patients with CD4 counts below 200 by substantially increasing HIV levels.

Cyclosporin

Cyclosporin has been used extensively to prevent tissue rejection in organ transplantation. Regarding its use in HIV treatment, *in vitro* experiments have demonstrated that it (i) suppresses T cell activation through the formation of cyclosporin-cyclophilin, a complex which inhibits the calcium and calmodulin-dependent protein phosphatase calcineurin. This prevents translocation of the transcription enhancer NFAT into the nucleus and results in a final block of activation of the genes for interleukin-2 (IL-2), the IL-2 receptor and IL-4 in T cells (Emmel et al., 1989); (ii) produces non-infectious HIV particles in chronically infected cells (Karpas et al., 1992); (iii) blocks the formation of syncytia – cellular aggregates which form around singly HIV-infected cells. Cyclosporin has also been used in primary HIV infection alongside HAART in order to restrict immune activation. A word of caution on cyclosporin is also necessary since it has been tried in the past and it is quite immune suppressive (Calabrese et al., 2002).

Conclusions

Even though HAART has substantially improved the prognosis for HIV-infected patients (in industrialized nations), there remains a dire need for cost-effective therapy in the developing countries, effective alternative maintenance therapy with a low resistance and toxicity profile, as well as new delivery modalities to simplify dosing schedules. This need will hopefully be met by therapeutic immunization or drugs which not only target the virus but also the debilitating hyperimmune activation. Immune reconstitution involves multiple novel mechanisms of action to impede HIV by targeting host cellular proteins that are not susceptible to mutation. Therefore, their resistance profile appears to be quite favorable. The induction of a potent HIV-specific cellular response through therapeutic immunization is now thought to be an attainable goal for HIV DNA vaccines.

Acknowledgements

The authors would like to thank Sylva Petrocchi for her editorial assistance.

References

Aichele P, Hengartner H, Zinkernagel RM, Schulz M. Antiviral cytotoxic T cell response induced by *in vivo* priming with a free synthetic peptide. J Exp Med 1990; 171: 1815–1820

Allison AC, Eugui EM. Mycophenolate mofetil and its mechanisms of action. Immunopharmacology 2000; 47: 85–118

Amara RR, Robinson HL. A new generation of HIV vaccines. Trends Mol Med 2002; 8: 489–495

Amara RR, Villinger F, Altman JD et al. Control of a mucosal challenge and prevention of AIDS by a multiprotein DNA/MVA vaccine. Science 2001; 292: 69–74

Ameisen JC, Capron A. Cell dysfunction and depletion in AIDS: the programmed cell death hypothesis. Immunol Today 1991; 12: 102–105

Andrieu M, Desoutter JF, Loing E et al. Two human immunodeficiency virus vaccinal lipopeptides follow different cross-presentation pathways in human dendritic cells. J Virol 2003; 77: 1564–1570

Barnett BG, Crews CJ, Douglas JT. Targeted adenoviral vectors. Biochim Biophys Acta 2002; 1575: 1–14

Barouch DH, Letvin NL. Viral evolution and challenges in the development of HIV vaccines. Vaccine 2002; 20 (Suppl 4): A66–68

Barouch DH, Santra S, Schmitz JE et al. Control of viremia and prevention of clinical AIDS in rhesus monkeys by cytokine-augmented DNA vaccination. Science 2000; 290: 486–492

Barouch DH, Kunstman J, Kuroda MJ et al. Eventual AIDS vaccine failure in a rhesus monkey by viral escape from cytotoxic T lymphocytes. Nature 2002; 415: 335–339

BenMohamed L, Wechsler SL, Nesburn AB. Lipopeptide vaccines – yesterday, today, and tomorrow. Lancet Infect Dis 2002; 2: 425–431

Bhardwaj N, Walker BD. Immunotherapy for AIDS virus infections: Cautious optimism for cell-based vaccine. Nat Med 2003; 9: 13–14

Calabrese LH, Lederman MM, Spritzler J et al. Placebo-controlled trial of cyclosporin-A in HIV-1 disease: implications for solid organ transplantation. J Acquir Immune Defic Syndr 2002; 29: 356–362

Chun TW, Engel D, Mizell SB et al. Effect of interleukin-2 on the pool of latently infected, resting CD4$^+$ T cells in HIV-1-infected patients receiving highly active antiretroviral therapy. Nat Med 1999; 5: 651–655

Colic M, Stojic-Vukanic Z, Pavlovic B, Jandric D, Stefanoska I. Mycophenolate mofetil inhibits differentiation, maturation and allostimulatory function of human monocyte-derived dendritic cells. Clin Exp Immunol 2003; 134: 63–69

De Boer RJ, Boucher CA, Perelson AS. Target cell availability and the successful suppression of HIV by hydroxyurea and didanosine. AIDS 1998; 12: 1567–1570

de Jong MD, Veenstra J, Stilianakis NI et al. Host-parasite dynamics and outgrowth of virus containing a single K70 R amino acid change in reverse transcriptase are responsible for the loss of human immunodeficiency virus type 1 RNA load suppression by zidovudine. Proc Natl Acad Sci USA 1996; 93: 5501–5506

Egan MA, Charini WA, Kuroda MJ et al. Simian immunodeficiency virus (SIV) gag DNA-vaccinated rhesus monkeys develop secondary cytotoxic T-lymphocyte responses and control viral replication after pathogenic SIV infection. J Virol 2000; 74: 7485–7495

Emmel EA, Verweij CL, Durand DB, Higgins KM, Lacy E, Crabtree GR. Cyclosporin A specifically inhibits function of nuclear proteins involved in T cell activation. Science 1989; 246: 1617–1620

Fayolle C, Deriaud E, Leclerc C. In vivo induction of cytotoxic T cell response by a free synthetic peptide requires CD4$^+$ T cell help. J Immunol 1991; 147: 4069–4073

Finkel TH, Tudor-Williams G, Banda NK et al. Apoptosis occurs predominantly in bystander cells and not in productively infected cells of HIV and SIV-infected lymph nodes. Nat Med 1995; 1: 129–134

Frieling U, Luger TA. Mycophenolate mofetil and leflunomide: promising compounds for the treatment of skin diseases. Clin Exp Dermatol 2002; 27: 562–570

Gao WY, Cara A, Gallo RC, Lori F. Low levels of deoxynucleotides in peripheral blood lymphocytes: a strategy to inhibit human immunodeficiency virus type 1 replication. Proc Natl Acad Sci USA 1993; 90: 8925–8928

Gao WY, Johns DG, Mitsuya H. Anti-human immunodeficiency virus type 1 activity of hydroxyurea in combination with 2', 3'-dideoxynucleosides. Mol Pharmacol 1994; 46: 767–772

Gao WY, Johns DG, Chokekuchai S, Mitsuya H. Disparate actions of hydroxyurea in potentiation of purine and pyrimidine 2', 3'-dideoxynucleoside activities against replication of a human immunodeficiency virus. Proc Natl Acad Sci USA 1995; 92: 8333–8337

Giorgi JV, Hultin LE, McKeating JA et al. Shorter survival in advanced human immunodeficiency virus type 1 infection is more closely associated with T lymphocyte activation than with plasma virus burden or virus chemokine coreceptor usage. J Infect Dis 1999; 179: 859–870

Gougeon ML, Lecoeur H, Dulioust A et al. Programmed cell death in peripheral lymphocytes from HIV-infected persons: increased susceptibility to apoptosis of CD4 and CD8 T cells correlates with lymphocyte activation and with disease progression. J Immunol 1996; 156: 3509–3520

Gupta K, Hudgens M, Corey L et al. Safety and immunogenicity of a high-titered canarypox vaccine in combination with rgp120 in a diverse population of HIV-1-uninfected adults: AIDS Vaccine Evaluation Group Protocol 022 A. J Acquir Immune Defic Syndr 2002; 29: 254–261

Hellerstein MK, Hoh RA, Hanley MB et al. Subpopulations of long-lived and short-lived T cells in advanced HIV-1 infection. J Clin Invest 2003; 112: 956–966

Heredia A, Amoroso A, Davis C et al. Rapamycin causes down-regulation of CCR5 and accumulation of anti-HIV beta-chemokines: an approach to suppress R5 strains of HIV-1. Proc Natl Acad Sci USA 2003; 100: 10411–10416

Jin X, Ramanathan Jr M, Barsoum S et al. Safety and immunogenicity of ALVAC vCP1452 and recombinant gp160 in newly human immunodeficiency virus type 1-infected patients treated with prolonged highly active antiretroviral therapy. J Virol 2002; 76: 2206–2216

Johns DG, Gao WY. Selective depletion of DNA precursors: an evolving strategy for potentiation of dideoxynucleoside activity against human immunodeficiency virus. Biochem Pharmacol 1998; 55: 1551–1556

Karpas A, Lowdell M, Jacobson SK, Hill F. Inhibition of human immunodeficiency virus and growth of infected T cells by the immunosuppressive drugs cyclosporin A and FK 506. Proc Natl Acad Sci USA 1992; 89: 8351–8355

Konno Y, Natsumeda Y, Nagai M et al. Expression of human IMP dehydrogenase types I and II in Escherichia coli and distribution in human normal lymphocytes and leukemic cell lines. J Biol Chem 1991; 266: 506–509

Korin YD, Zack JA. Progression to the G1 b phase of the cell cycle is required for completion of human immunodeficiency virus type 1 reverse transcription in T cells. J Virol 1998; 72: 3161–3168

Lisziewicz J, Rosenberg E, Lieberman J et al. Control of HIV despite the discontinuation of antiretroviral therapy. N Engl J Med 1999; 340: 1683–1684

Lisziewicz J, Bakare N, Lori F. Therapeutic vaccination for future management of HIV/AIDS. Vaccine 2003; 21: 620–623

Lisziewicz J, Trocio J, Whitman L et al. Derma Vir: a novel topical vaccine for HIV/AIDS. J Invest Dermatol 2005a; 124: 160–169

Lisziewicz J, Trocio J, Xu J e tal. Control of viral rebound through therapeutic immunization with Derma Vir. AIDS 2005b; 19: 35–43

Lori F. Hydroxyurea and HIV: 5 years later – from antiviral to immune-modulating effects. AIDS 1999; 13: 1433–1442

Lori F, Lisziewicz J. Cellular factors: targets for the treatment of HIV infection. Antivir Ther 1998; 3 (Suppl 4): 81–92

Lori F, Lisziewicz J. Structured treatment interruptions for the management of HIV infection. JAMA 2001; 286: 2981–2987

Lori F, Malykh A, Cara A et al. Hydroxyurea as an inhibitor of human immunodeficiency virus-type 1 replication. Science 1994; 266: 801–805

Lori F, Lewis MG, Xu J et al. Control of SIV rebound through structured treatment interruptions during early infection. Science 2000; 290: 1591–1593

Lu W, Wu X, Lu Y, Guo W, Andrieu JM. Therapeutic dendritic-cell vaccine for simian AIDS. Nat Med 2003; 9: 27–32

Lui SL, Ramassar V, Urmson J, Halloran PF. Mycophenolate mofetil reduces production of interferon-dependent major histocompatibility complex induction during allograft rejection, probably by limiting clonal expansion. Transpl Immunol 1998; 6: 23–32

MacGregor RR, Ginsberg R, Ugen KE et al. T-cell responses induced in normal volunteers immunized with a DNA-based vaccine containing HIV-1 env and rev. AIDS 2002; 16: 2137–2143

Malley SD, Grange JM, Hamedi-Sangsari F, Vila JR. Suppression of HIV production in resting lymphocytes by combining didanosine and hydroxamate compounds. Lancet 1994; 343: 1292

Margolis D, Heredia A, Gaywee J, Oldach D, Drusano G, Redfield R. Abacavir and mycophenolic acid, an inhibitor of inosine monophosphate dehydrogenase, have profound and synergistic anti-HIV activity. J Acquir Immune Defic Syndr 1999; 21: 362–370

McAdam AJ, Gewurz BE, Farkash EA, Sharpe AH. Either B7 costimulation or IL-2 can elicit generation of primary alloreactive CTL. J Immunol 2000; 165: 3088–3093

McLean AR, Emery VC, Webster A, Griffiths PD. Population dynamics of HIV within an individual after treatment with zidovudine. AIDS 1991; 5: 485–489

McLean AR, Nowak MA. Competition between zidovudine-sensitive and zidovudine-resistant strains of HIV. AIDS 1992; 6: 71–79

Meyaard L, Otto SA, Jonker RR, Mijnster MJ, Keet RP, Miedema F. Programmed death of T cells in HIV-1 infection. Science 1992; 257: 217–219

Nagai M, Natsumeda Y, Weber G. Proliferation-linked regulation of type II IMP dehydrogenase gene in human normal lymphocytes and HL-60 leukemic cells. Cancer Res 1992; 52: 258–261

Natarajan V, Lempicki RA, Sereti I et al. Increased peripheral expansion of naive CD4+ T cells in vivo after IL-2 treatment of patients with HIV infection. Proc Natl Acad Sci USA 2002; 99: 10712–10717

Ourmanov I, Brown CR, Moss B et al. Comparative efficacy of recombinant modified vaccinia virus Ankara expressing simian immunodeficiency virus (SIV) Gag-Pol and/or Env in macaques challenged with pathogenic SIV. J Virol 2000; 74: 2740–2751

Paiardini M, Galati D, Cervasi B et al. Exogenous interleukin-2 administration corrects the cell cycle perturbation of lymphocytes from human immunodeficiency virus-infected individuals. J Virol 2001; 75: 10843–10855

Palmer S, Shafer RW, Merigan TC. Hydroxyurea enhances the activities of didanosine, 9-(2-[phosphonylmethoxy]ethyl) adenine, and 9-(2-[phosphonylmethoxy]propyl) adenine against drug-susceptible and drug-resistant human immunodeficiency virus

isolates. Antimicrob Agents Chemother 1999; 43: 2046–2050

Phillips AN. Reduction of HIV concentration during acute infection: independence from a specific immune response. Science 1996; 271: 497–499

Pialoux G, Gahery-Segard H, Sermet S et al. Lipopeptides induce cell-mediated anti-HIV immune responses in seronegative volunteers. AIDS 2001; 15: 1239–1249

Piazza P, Fan Z, Rinaldo Jr CR. CD8+ T-cell immunity to HIV infection. Clin Lab Med 2002; 22: 773–797

Puaux AL, Michel ML. New gene-based approaches for an AIDS vaccine. Comp Immunol Microbiol Infect Dis 2003; 26: 357–372

Rosenberg ES, Altfeld M, Poon SH et al. Immune control of HIV-1 after early treatment of acute infection. Nature 2000; 407: 523–526

Rossio JL, Esser MT, Suryanarayana K et al. Inactivation of human immunodeficiency virus type 1 infectivity with preservation of conformational and functional integrity of virion surface proteins. J Virol 1998; 72: 7992–8001

Rowland-Jones SL. HIV: The deadly passenger in dendritic cells. Curr Biol 1999; 9: R248–250

Shiver JW, Fu TM, Chen L et al. Replication-incompetent adenoviral vaccine vector elicits effective anti-immunodeficiency-virus immunity. Nature 2002; 415: 331–335

Singh M, O'Hagan D. Advances in vaccine adjuvants. Nat Biotechnol 1999; 17: 1075–1081

Sopper S, Nierwetberg D, Halbach A et al. Impact of simian immunodeficiency virus (SIV) infection on lymphocyte numbers and T-cell turnover in different organs of rhesus monkeys. Blood 2003; 101: 1213–1219

Sousa AE, Carneiro J, Meier-Schellersheim M, Grossman Z, Victorino RM. CD4 T cell depletion is linked directly to immune activation in the pathogenesis of HIV-1 and HIV-2 but only indirectly to the viral load. J Immunol 2002; 169: 3400–3406

Stevenson M, Stanwick TL, Dempsey MP, Lamonica CA. HIV-1 replication is controlled at the level of T cell activation and proviral integration. The Embo Journal 1990; 9: 1551–1560

Wein LM, D'Amato RM, Perelson AS. Mathematical analysis of antiretroviral therapy aimed at HIV-1 eradication or maintenance of low viral loads. J Theor Biol 1998; 192: 81–98

Zack JA, Arrigo SJ, Weitsman SR, Go AS, Haislip A, Chen IS. HIV-1 entry into quiescent primary lymphocytes: molecular analysis reveals a labile, latent viral structure. Cell 1990; 61: 213–222

Zinkernagel RM, Hengartner H. T-cell-mediated immunopathology versus direct cytolysis by virus: implications for HIV and AIDS. Immunol Today 1994; 15: 262–268

2.2 Long-Term Control of HIV-1 RNA Replication Following a Unique STI and Mycophenolate Mofetil Therapy in Patients Treated with HAART Since PHI

G. Tambussi

Introduction

When to start antiretroviral therapy, particularly in symptomatic HIV-1-infected subjects with primary HIV infection (PHI), is currently being extensively debated. Early intervention with highly active antiretroviral therapy (HAART) during PHI has been shown to augment the HIV-specific T helper response that is similar only in long-term non-progressors, although the effects on the magnitude and persistence of the cytotoxic T-lymphocyte (CTL) response during PHI have not yet been well defined.

Nevertheless, the inability of HAART to achieve eradication of HIV-1, along with the emerging issues of long-term toxicities associated with a lifelong commitment to therapy, calls for the development of alternative therapeutic strategies in patients who have been treated during PHI. One of the conceivable approaches aimed at achieving long-term control of the virus, even when antiviral therapy is simplified or temporarily definitely discontinued, is the so-called structured/supervised treatment interruption (STI). In the last years many reports have suggested the usefulness of STI after a long period of complete virus suppression.

The development of such strategies has encountered some crucial problems. In particular, the initiation of HAART is followed by a relative increase in the proportion of cells that are active and/or proliferating (Rosenberg et al., 1997), thus being able to support new rounds of infection and virus production (Ho, 1998). This consideration, together with the emergence of drug-resistance virus strains that usually further complicated the correct use of such strategies, emphasizes the need to test alternative therapeutic options.

Among these, immune-based interventions which include antiretroviral drugs in combination with compounds that are able to modulate the function and reactivity of the immune system might be pursued. The goal of these modalities is to achieve long-term control of virus replication with a minimal or possibly no use of antiretroviral drugs. In this context, it is worth exploring the potential use of immune-modulating drugs, such as mycophenolic acid that, on account of their mechanism of action, may also exert an antiviral activity.

Mycophenolate mofetil (MMF) is a well-known drug which is broadly used in renal transplantation for its ability to selectively inhibit lymphocyte division. MMF is the morpholinoethyl ester of the active compound mycophenolic acid (MPA). Interest in MMF as an immunosuppressive agent in renal transplantation has been renewed by clinical studies showing that the proliferation of T and B lymphocytes is selectively blocked by MPA because their purine synthesis primarily relies on the *de novo* synthesis pathway which is blocked by MPA.

The effect of MMF on cell activation and HIV-1 infection has been investigated in both *in vitro* and *in vivo* animal studies. Overall, available data indicate that MMF is a potent inhibitor of the proliferation of activated T cells, even in the presence of IL-2, and suppresses cell proliferation by inducing apoptosis and cell death of a large proportion of activated T cells. These results suggest that MMF might be able to significantly reduce the size of the pool of dividing $CD4^+$ T cells *in vivo* (Chapuis et al., 2000). An open question is whether or not MMF exerts an effect on the pool of resting latently infected $CD4^+$ T cells. It is likely that MMF has no effect on a resting cell, and thus it does not affect directly the size of this pool of cells. However, once these cells are activated in the presence of MMF, MMF might in turn induce apoptosis and therefore cell death. Taken together, these preliminary data suggest that MMF might have an indirect impact on the pool of resting, latently infected $CD4^+$ T cells, contributing to its depletion *in vivo*.

Moreover, abacavir (ABC) and MMF are highly synergistic in reducing virus load (Coull et al.,

2001; Margolis et al., 2002; Press et al., 2002), nearly 8fold more synergistic than the effect reported for the combination of ABC and amprenavir. The IC_{50} value for MPA is 0.1 µM, 10- to 100fold below the trough levels seen clinically in organ transplant patients. In the presence or absence of ABC, 0.25 µM MPA had little effect on cell proliferation.

The aim of this pilot, non-randomized study was to assess whether the combined use of a unique supervised treatment interruption (USTI) and MMF in patients successfully treated during PHI is able or not to interfere with the dynamics of viral rebound, and ultimately with the kinetics of the immune response, usually seen soon after the interruption of an active antiretroviral therapy.

Patients

Since the onset of PHI, 14 patients have been treated with HAART for 4.9 ± 0.8 (mean ± SD) years, all achieving optimal suppression of VL for 3.6 ± 0.7 years. Before USTI, all patients had added MMF 500 mg bid to HAART at week − 2. At week 0 HAART was stopped and MMF 500 mg QD was continued for 24 weeks.

Patients of the USTI/MMF group received a 2-week induction MMF/HAART-(ART) regimen. At the end of this period all subjects stopped antiretroviral therapy, while MMF was continued. Conventional HAART (ABC/1 RTI/1 or 2 protease inhibitors [PIs]) was restarted when plasma viral load exceeded 100,000 copies/mL (100 Kcp/mL) verified on at least 2 consecutive tests.

As controls, 6 well-matched PHI patients on HAART for 2.7 ± 0.2 years and with suppressed VL for 2.3 ± 0.1 years underwent USTI without MMF. Plasma VL was measured with the Nasba-Organon assay (limit of detection: 80 copies/mL).

Antiretroviral Therapy Prior to STI

Due to the length of the antiretroviral therapy prior to the enrolment into the study (at least 48 weeks of HAART), the patients at the time of enrolment could be treated with non-homogeneous schemes of therapy, i.e., containing ABC and PIs or not. In order to exploit the potential synergistic effect described for the combination MMF/ABC, the only mandatory antiretroviral drug at the time of the enrolment must be considered as ABC.

Use of Potential Drugs which Antagonize MMF

Some *in vitro* data seem to suggest a potential antagonistic effect between zidovudine and stavudine and MMF. When possible, these drugs have been stopped and changed with other antiretroviral agents, but this modification of the ongoing therapy was not mandatory.

Results

All patients have been followed for at least 78 weeks. The matrix below (Fig. 2.**3**) shows each VL determination in the MMF group over time depicted in varying colors according to VL categories.

Following USTI and MMF, 11 of 14 patients have maintained a very effective VL control over time, mostly < 5 Kcp/mL, along with stable or decreasing levels of HIV-1 DNA, and slightly decreasing $CD4^+$ T cell counts (week 0: mean ± SD, 1020 ± 266 cells/mL; week 48: 805 ± 185).

Only 3 of 14 patients (Nos. 12 − 14) discontinued MMF and restarted HAART, achieving optimal VL control and increasing $CD4^+$ T cell counts over week 0.

In contrast, 4 of 6 controls restarted HAART within the first 12 weeks after USTI (Fig. 2.**4**), and the remaining 2 controls had VL of 35 and 5 Kcp/mL, respectively, with a substantial decrease in $CD4^+$ T cell counts at week 48 (− 444 and − 373 cells/mL over week 0, respectively).

Of note, rebound VL slopes were significantly lower in the 14 MMF patients than in controls (slope to the highest VL value: + 755 vs. + 10 214 cp/mL/day, respectively, p = 0.03; slope to week 4: + 657 vs. + 12 098 cp/mL/day, respectively, p = 0.01).

Looking at the CD4 dynamics in responder patients after stopping therapy, in the USTI/MMF group CD4 T cell counts remained substantially stable during the first 24 weeks of treatment, while slight decreases have been observed from week 24 and week 78 (Fig. 2.**5**).

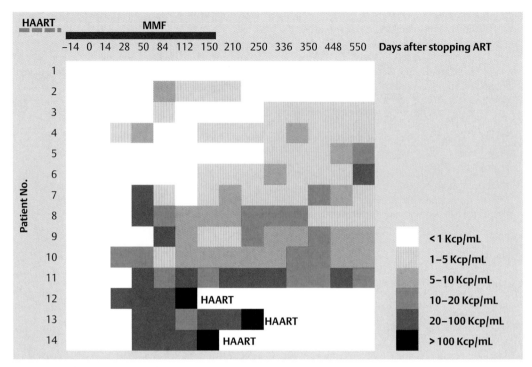

Fig. 2.**3**   VL determinations in the MMF group over time.

Conclusions

The advent of HAART has radically changed the clinical course of HIV infection. However, recent advances in the pathogenesis of the infection, including the analysis of T cell dynamic changes induced by the virus and HIV-1 cellular reservoirs (Finzi et al., 1997; Chun et al., 1997), emphasize the fact that HIV-1 eradication is not likely to occur, even following a life-long use of effective antiretroviral therapy.

The inability of HAART to achieve eradication of HIV-1 along with the emerging issues of long-term toxicities associated with a life-long commitment to therapy also calls for the development of alternative therapeutic strategies aimed at achieving long-term control of the virus even when antiviral therapy is simplified or temporarily or definitely discontinued.

The potential usefulness of supervised treatment interruption and MMF in patient successfully treated during PHI has been explored in this pilot study in order to assess whether or not this approach is able to interfere with the dynamics of viral rebound, and ultimately with the kinetics of the immune response, usually seen soon after the interruption of an active antiretroviral therapy.

Unlike STI alone, the combination of USTI and 24 weeks of MMF is associated with a long-term control of virus replication in more than 75% of the cases. Regarding CD4 cell count dynamics, three distinct phases have been observed: 1) soon after the introduction of the induction therapy with MMF 550 mg BID a decrease of CD4 occurs; 2) interestingly, this decay is not worsened by the subsequent 24 weeks of halved dose of MMF; 3) a slight progressive decrease of CD4 is observed from week 24 to week 78. This phenomenon clearly deserves further investigations.

In patients who did have a significant outbreak of viral replication after stopping therapy, a prompt response to new HAART in terms of recovery of circulating CD4 T lymphocytes and decay of viral load was observed. This could suggest that the use of MMF in the context of STI does not negatively affect the efficacy of a subsequent use of an effective antiretroviral therapy. It should be noted that no major side effects related to the study drug have been observed.

Studies on changes in pathogen-specific helper and cytotoxic effector T cells are currently being performed.

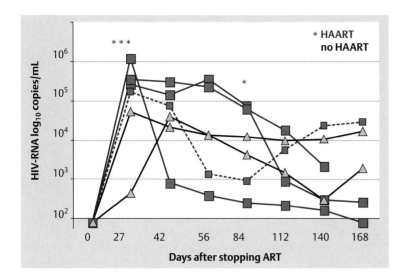

Fig. 2.**4** VL control over time following USTI and MMF.

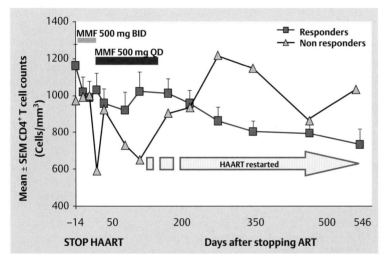

Fig. 2.**5** CD4 dynamics in responder patients in the USTI/MMF group after stopping therapy.

References

Chapuis A, Paolo Rizzardi G, D'Agostino C et al. Effects of mycophenolic acid on human immunodeficiency virus infection *in vitro* and *in vivo*. Nat Med 2000; 6: 762–768

Chun TW, Stuyver L, Mizell SB et al. Presence of an inducible HIV-1 latent reservoir during highly active antiretroviral therapy. Proc Natl Acad Sci USA 1997; 94: 13193–13197

Coull JJ, Turner D, Melby T et al. A pilot study of the use of mycophenolate mofetil as a component of therapy for multidrug-resistant HIV-1 infection. J Acquir Immune Defic Syndr 2001; 26: 423–434

Finzi D, Hermankova M, Pierson T et al. Identification of a reservoir for HIV 1 in patients on highly active antiretroviral therapy. Science 1997; 278: 1295–1300

Ho DD. Toward HIV eradication or remission: the tasks ahead. Science 1998; 280: 1866–1867

Margolis DM, Kewn S, Coull JJ et al. The addition of mycophenolate mofetil to antiretroviral therapy including abacavir is associated with depletion of intracellular deoxyguanosine triphosphate and a decrease in plasma HIV-1 RNA. J Acquir Immune Defic Syndr 2002; 31: 45–49

Press N, Kimel G, Harris M et al. Case series assessing the safety of mycophenolate as part of multidrug rescue treatment regimens. HIV Clin Trials 2002; 3: 17–20

Rosenberg ES, Billingsley JM, Caliendo AM et al. Vigorous HIV-1 specific CD4+ T cell responses associated with control of viremia. Science 1997; 278: 1447–1450

2.3 Supervised Treatment Interruptions in Acute HIV Infection

D. E. Kaufmann, B. D. Walker

Introduction

The use of highly active antiretroviral therapy (HAART) can significantly prolong the life of individuals infected by human immunodeficiency virus 1 (HIV-1) (Palella et al., 1998), but early hopes for virus eradication have not come to fruition (Finzi et al., 1999). The successful use of HAART is limited by drug-related toxicities, high costs, and drug resistance (Richman, 2001), factors that have led to the development of alternative therapeutic strategies. Mounting evidence indicates that viral control and disease progression are influenced by HIV-1-specific immune responses. Therefore, an alternative approach to lifelong treatment may be to develop immune-based therapies with the goal of generating adequate immune responses that will control HIV-1 in the absence of HAART (Allen et al., 2002). The concept of immune boosting through supervised, or structured, treatment interruption (STI) was introduced first through reports of anecdotal cases (Lisziewicz et al., 1999; Lori et al., 1999; Ortiz et al., 1999) and later through limited and non-controlled clinical trials (Rosenberg et al., 2000). The rationale of this approach is based on the observation that new naïve cells are generated under HAART (Autran et al., 1997) and that recurrent limited exposure to autologous virus might prime these cells to target HIV-1. This approach has been unsuccessful in chronic infection (Oxenius et al., 2002; Fagard et al., 2003 b), but has been shown to lead to at least transient containment of viremia after intervention in the acute phase of infection in humans and animals exposed to AIDS-associated retroviruses (Lori et al., 2000; Rosenberg et al., 2000; Markowitz et al., 2002).

We present here the results of a study (Kaufmann et al., 2004) in which we performed an in-depth longitudinal analysis of the impact of early treatment followed by STIs in patients treated during acute or early HIV-1 infection and discuss it in the perspective of other STI trials. The central hypothesis of the study was that early treatment of acute HIV-1 infection would induce immunologic maturation and subsequent effective control of HIV-1 without the need for continual drug therapy. Alternatively, if a breakthrough of virus replication was observed, this strategy would lead to exposure to viral antigen and thereby result in an increase in HIV-1-specific immunity after reinstitution of antiviral therapy. The primary endpoint was the time to viral rebound above 50,000 copies/mL once or above 5,000 copies for three separate visits, each a week apart. The secondary goal was to correlate immunologic and virologic parameters with any observed effects including evolution of HIV-1-specific cellular immune responses. The early results of this trial were previously reported, showing that five of eight patients were able to reach a plasma viral load of 500 copies/mL or less at a median of 6 months off therapy (Rosenberg et al., 2000). The current study investigated the frequency and resilience of control achieved with this intervention, with follow-up to a median of 5.3 years post-infection, and with an increased cohort size of 14 patients. Our results indicate that, although the majority of patients treated in the acute phase of infection go on to control HIV-1 to less than 5000 RNA copies/mL plasma for at least 6 months off therapy, the ability to contain viremia at or below this level for an extended period of time is uncommon.

Study Population and STIs

Fourteen patients presenting with acute or early HIV-1 infection were enrolled in this study between July 1997 and January 2000. All participants in the study had symptoms congruent with an acute retroviral syndrome and were treated with HAART (one protease inhibitor and two nucleoside reverse transcriptase inhibitors) within a median of 19 days after onset of symptoms. The median viral load at the start of therapy was 515,000 RNA copies/mL plasma (range: 5500 to 9,600,000). Patients underwent successive treatment interruptions after successful initial treatment of at least 8 months. After a treatment interruption, patients were closely monitored and therapy was restarted if viral load remained above 5000 RNA copies/mL plasma for longer than three consecutive weeks, or was in excess of 50,000 copies/mL on any single occasion.

Table 2.1 Period of viral control achieved off therapy

Duration of Viral Control (days)	Number of Patients
90	11/14
180	8/14
270	7/14
360	6/14
540	5/14
>720	3/14

Longitudinal Assessment of Control of Viremia Following Treated Acute or Early Infection

The fourteen patients entered into this protocol were followed for a median of 5.3 years from the time of infection (range: 494–2475 days). For purposes of analysis, patients who dropped out of the study or who restarted therapy without meeting criteria were regarded as having lost the ability to contain viremia.

Using these criteria for re-initiation of therapy and to define failure, 11 of 14 patients (79%) were able to achieve virologic control to less than 5000 RNA copies/mL plasma for at least 90 days after one, two, or three treatment interruptions (Table 2.1), supporting the earlier observations in the smaller cohort. The period of longest containment was after one interruption for five patients, after two interruptions for eight patients, and after three interruptions for one patient (Table 2.2). Six of 14 patients (43%) controlled viremia for one year after stopping therapy, but only three of 14 (21%) were able to control viremia off therapy at

Table 2.2 Time to failure during the STIs

Patient	Number of STI Cycles	Time to Failure or Last Follow-Up (Days)[a]		
		First STI	Second STI	Third STI
AC-10	1	1346[b]		
AC-15	1	666		
AC-45	1	71		
AC-02	2	10	1351[b]	
AC-13	2	90[c]	270[c]	
AC-16	2	561	35	
AC-33	2	366	222	
AC-14	3	35	147	1070
AC-25	3	35	49	37
AC-26	3	35	47	42
AC-46	3	104	158	96
AC-04	4	50	167	37
AC-05	4	21	121[c]	45
AC-06	4	61	310[d]	21
Median (range)	66 (10–1346)	158 (35–1351)	42 (21–1070)	

[a] Numbers correspond to time until virological failure, unless otherwise specified. Shaded gray indicates the longest time off therapy until failure or last follow-up.
[b] Last follow-up visit; patient still meeting criteria of virological control.
[c] Failure because patient restarted antiviral therapy without meeting criteria of virological failure.
[d] Virological failure due to HIV-1 superinfection.

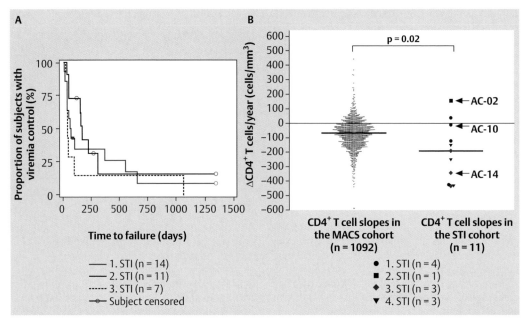

Fig. 2.**6 a, b**   Evolution of viral load and CD4⁺ T cell count during STI. **a** Survival curves of time to virologic failure during the first three supervised treatment interruptions. Virologic failure was defined as having a viral load of greater than 5000 copies RNA/mL plasma for 3 weeks or greater than 50,000 copies once. Patients still achieving viral control at the last visit and individuals restarting therapy without meeting criteria or lost to follow-up are censored at the last evaluable time point. The horizontal axis represents the time off therapy since the beginning of the treatment interruption, the vertical axis corresponds to the number of patients maintaining control of viremia. The curves for first, second, and third STIs do not differ significantly from each other (log-rank test, $p > 0.05$). **b** Evolution of CD4⁺ T cell counts during the longest treatment interruption. Slopes of CD4⁺ T cell counts during the first year of the longest treatment interruption are shown for patients who experienced a cessation of therapy of at least 12 months (all except AC-13, AC-25, and AC-45), compared to the natural decline of CD4⁺ T cell counts in untreated patients of the MACS cohort with early chronic HIV-1 infection (CD4⁺ counts of > 350 cells/mm³). CD4⁺ T cell losses were calculated on a regression line based on least squares fit. The two groups differed significantly from each other (Mann-Whitney U test, $p = 0.02$).

less than 5000 RNA copies/mL plasma for more than 2 years. Duration of viremia control during successive treatment interruptions was highly variable, and there was no increase in the sustainability of viral containment during successive STI cycles. The three patients achieving control of viremia for more than 2 years did so during the first (AC-10), the second (AC-02), and the third (AC-14) treatment interruption, respectively (Fig. 2.**6 a**). A paired comparison (Wilcoxon matched-pairs signed-ranks test) showed no significant difference in the length of viremia control with subsequent treatment interruptions. Although patients experienced rebound viremia after discontinuing therapy, none of the patients experienced reappearance of symptoms associated with acute HIV-1 infection.

These data show that at least transient control of viremia to less than 5000 RNA copies/mL plasma was achieved in the majority of study participants during at least one of the treatment interruptions. However, durable viral control in participants following treated acute infection occurred infrequently. Moreover, the data do not show a pattern of better viral control with sequential treatment interruptions.

Effect of Treatment Interruptions on CD4⁺ T Cell Counts

Although viral load is a strong predictor of disease progression, CD4⁺ T cell loss is an additional, independent predictor (Cozzi Lepri et al., 1998). Early treatment of acute HIV-1 infection led to normalization of CD4$^+$ T cell counts in most patients, but the effect of treatment interruption was variable, even in those doing well, as defined by sustained low viremia. Overall, 11 of 14 patients interrupted therapy for at least 12 months and these individuals were evaluated with respect to the effect of treatment interruption on CD4^1 T cell loss (Fig. 2.**6b**). The rate of change in CD4$^+$ T cell counts during the first year of the longest period off treatment ranged from + 157 to – 438 cells/mm^3/year (median: – 192). Of the three patients who did not meet viral load criteria for restarting therapy for more than 2 years, one (AC-02) had an increasing CD4$^+$ T cell count of 157 cells/mm^3/year, one (AC-10) had a stable CD4$^+$ T cell count (– 9 cells/mm^3/year), and one (AC-14) experienced a loss of 344 cells/mm^3/year. Comparison with data from the Multicenter AIDS Cohort Study (MACS) showed that the kinetics of CD4$^+$ T cell decline was faster (Mann-Whitney U test, $p = 0.02$) than in untreated patients with early chronic HIV-1 infection (average loss of – 67 cells/mm^3/year in patients with a CD4$^+$ T cell count of more than 350 cells/mm^3 at baseline). However, the CD4$^+$ T cell loss rate was comparable to what has been described after treatment interruption in chronic HIV-1 infection (Tebas et al., 2002; Maggiolo et al., 2004). These results denote that periods of relative control of viremia were associated with declining CD4$^+$ T cell counts in most patients.

Correlation of Clinical and Genetic Markers with Duration of Viremia Control

Although the study was small, we evaluated clinical and laboratory parameters to see if any were predictive of duration of viral control. Analyses included clinical and laboratory data at the time of presentation with acute HIV-1 infection, genetic markers associated with different rates of disease progression, and the presence or absence of GBV-C coinfection. All patients presented with symptomatic acute infection. Time between onset of symptoms and institution of therapy did not affect duration of control following STI (Cox proportional hazards regression model, $p > 0.05$). The individuals who controlled viremia for a longer period during any of the treatment interruptions were not different from those who experienced earlier breakthrough as measured by ELISA and Western blot status at initiation of HAART, coreceptor polymorphisms (CCR5delta32, CCR2 V64I), or the presence or absence of GBV-C coinfection (Cox proportional hazards model, $p > 0.05$ in all comparisons). The only parameter that was predictive of prolonged viral control during the first treatment interruption was a low viremia at the time of institution of therapy ($p = 0.01$): there was a 2.8fold increase in hazard per order of magnitude increase in viral load. This factor was no longer predictive when the period of longest control of viremia was taken into account. The time to rebound of viremia (> 50 copies/mL or > 400 copies/mL) did not correlate with the duration of viral control. Although 11 out of 14 individuals achieved at least transient control of viremia, and three experienced prolonged control, none of these patients possessed the HLA alleles B27 or B57, associated with better disease outcome (Kaslow et al., 1996; Migueles et al., 2000).

Relationship of Magnitude and Breadth of HIV-1-Specific T Cell Responses to Duration of Viremia Control

To evaluate the relationship between the clinical outcome and evolution of HIV-1-specific CD8$^+$ T cells, we longitudinally analyzed the breadth and magnitude of CD8$^+$ T cell responses using an interferon-γ ELISPOT assay and overlapping peptides spanning the entire HIV-1 clade B consensus sequence (Fig. 2.**7**). At the beginning of the first STI, HIV-1-specific CD8$^+$ T cells were weak and narrowly directed at a median of two epitopes. CD8$^+$ T cell responses increased significantly ($p < 0.05$) during the first off-treatment period, and remained when therapy was reintroduced. A further increase in the magnitude and breadth of HIV-1-specific CD8$^+$ T cells was observed in the subsequent off-treatment periods, although these augmentations failed to reach statistical significance. The CD8$^+$ T cell-mediated immune responses emerging during these consecutive cycles of treatment interruption were broadly directed, targeting all structural and most accessory and regulatory HIV-1 gene products. However, the magnitude of HIV-1-specific CD8$^+$ T cell responses at the beginning of the successive treatment interruptions was not predictive of the time the study participants were subsequently able to stay off therapy.

We next analyzed evolution of lymphoproliferative responses to recombinant HIV-1 p24 Gag protein in order to assess HIV-1-specific CD4$^+$ T cell function. Most individuals had no detectable response at baseline prior to treatment, consistent

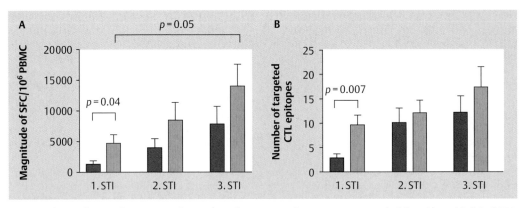

Fig. 2.**7 a, b**   Evolution of HIV-1-specific CD8[+] T cell responses during STI. Magnitude (**a**) and breadth (**b**) of HIV-specific CD8[+] responses on the first day of treatment interruption (red bars) and on the last day off therapy (grey bars). Data represent the mean and standard deviation. PBMC = peripheral blood mononuclear cells; SFC = spot-forming cells.

with prior studies on acute HIV-1 infection (Rosenberg et al., 1997). After initiation of HAART, all individuals generated HIV-1-specific lymphoproliferative responses, which was a criterion for inclusion in the study. During treatment interruptions, there was a variable decline in magnitude. Similar to CD8[+] T cell responses, the magnitude of HIV-1-specific CD4[+] T helper cell responses at the beginning of the treatment interruptions was not statistically predictive of the time the study participants were subsequently able to stay off therapy according to study criteria.

Discussion

Early treatment of acute HIV-1 infection followed by treatment interruptions may enhance control of viremia (Rosenberg et al., 2000), but the durability of this control has been uncertain. Here we analyzed the long-term effects of initiation of antiviral therapy during acute HIV-1 infection followed by STIs in a cohort of 14 patients. Although initial control of viremia to less than 5000 RNA copies/mL plasma was achieved in the majority of the individuals studied, a gradual increase in viremia and decline in CD4[+] T cell counts were observed in most patients. Durable virologic control was not frequent, despite the presence of robust HIV-1-specific CD4[+] and CD8[+] T cell responses detected by standard assays. Moreover, even during periods of successful viral control, progressive loss of CD4[+] T cells was frequently observed. These data indicate that, although early treatment of acute and

early infection is frequently associated with transient control of viremia after STI, ongoing low-level viral replication is associated with eventual virologic breakthrough in most patients.

The standard immunologic assays and virologic assessments in this cohort showed considerable heterogeneity among the study participants, and did not show a consistent pattern in duration of viremia control during successive treatment interruptions. Eleven of 14 patients (79%) were able to maintain a viral load of less than 5000 copies/mL for at least 90 days, but progressive loss of control was common in the majority of patients and only three patients (21%) were able to maintain control for more than 2 years. Clinical, genetic, and immunological parameters did not distinguish these three individuals from the other 11 patients, nor did they predict the duration of control following treatment interruption. Indeed, the longer a patient was off therapy, the stronger and more broadly directed the CD8[+] T cell responses became, but these were insufficient to maintain prolonged control in most patients.

Loss of viral control in this cohort occurred not only in the presence of strong CD8[+] T cell responses, but in most cases also in the presence of virus-specific CD4[+] T cell responses, although the CD4[+] T cell responses were observed to decline during periods of viremia. In addition, total CD4[+] T cell numbers were also followed, and declined in most patients over time, including one of the three patients who were able to suppress viremia for at least 2 years. Mechanisms leading to rapid CD4[+] T cell loss need to be further studied in future STI trials. Other parameters including chemokine receptor polymorphisms (Dean et al., 1996) and GBV-C coinfection (Tillmann et al., 2001; Xiang et al., 2001) similarly failed to explain the variety of courses following treatment interruption. The only parameter found to be associated with longer control of viremia during the first treatment interruption was a lower viral load at the time of institution of antiviral therapy. Given the multiplicity of comparisons made, the true significance of this finding is uncertain.

The reasons for progressive loss of control despite augmentation of virus-specific CD4$^+$ and CD8$^+$ T cell responses are yet to be defined. In one individual (AC-06), HIV-1 superinfection in the setting of strong and broadly directed HIV-specific cellular immune responses was associated with the loss of viral control, as previously reported (Altfeld et al., 2002). No other cases of superinfection have been identified in these patients. The immunologic studies performed failed to show an association between increases in viral load and loss of immune responses, but this may be due to the use of the current standard IFN-γ assays to measure immune function. Numerous studies now indicate that IFN-γ production alone is not associated with viral load (Betts et al., 2001; Addo et al., 2003; Draenert et al., 2004) but rather that functional characteristics of CD4$^+$ and CD8$^+$ T cells may be better associated with viral control (Migueles et al., 2002; Wherry et al., 2003a; Wherry et al., 2003b; Lichterfeld et al., 2004a). Such studies will be important to pursue. Full evaluation of the relationship between immune escape and viral breakthrough will require extensive additional analyses in future studies, including detailed analysis of responses to autologous virus (Lee et al., 2002; Altfeld et al., 2003).

It is important to view these findings in the light of other recent data on treatment interruption in both acute and chronic infection. In chronic HIV-1 infection, STI studies showed only marginal, if any, improvements of HIV-1 viremia control following a number of treatment interruption cycles, despite at least transient increases in HIV-1-specific CD8$^+$ and CD4$^+$ T cell responses (Carcelain et al., 2001; Ortiz et al., 2001; Oxenius et al., 2002; Fagard et al., 2003b). In the setting of infection with a multidrug-resistant virus, this strategy may even be harmful (Lawrence et al., 2003). Other studies of STI after treated acute HIV-1 infection have shown limited benefits (Markowitz et al., 2002), including recent trials such as the PrimSTOP trial (Hoen et al., 2004) and the QUEST study (Kinloch

et al., 2004). However, not enough is known about the relationship between scheduling of HAART and treatment interruptions and the characteristics of viral rebound after therapy has been stopped.

Although durable control of viremia was not achieved, the majority of patients were able to sustain transient containment of viremia, suggesting that future studies aimed at further enhancing immune control may be warranted. Early treatment alone should still be considered an important avenue for therapy. Therapeutic vaccinations administered after treated acute HIV-1 infection and before cessation of therapy have thus far given disappointing results (Markowitz et al., 2002), but the design of new and more potent immunogens requires reassessment of this approach. Indeed, the ability to enhance CD4$^+$ T helper cell responses in the chronic phase of infection has been demonstrated (Robbins et al., 2003), and this effect has been shown to correlate with enhanced HIV-specific CD8$^+$ T cell proliferative capacity in response to viral antigens *in vitro* (Lichterfeld et al., 2004b). Some promising results have been achieved using immunomodulatory drugs, including cyclosporine (Rizzardi et al., 2002) and hydroxyurea (Lafeuillade et al., 2003), in combination with antiviral therapy, presumably because of the limitation of T cell activation. Administration of granulocyte-macrophage colony-stimulating factor stunted the viral rebound following interruption of HAART, and largely prevented a decrease of CD4$^+$ T cell counts in an STI trial in chronic HIV-1 infection (Fagard et al. 2003a). These additional therapeutic interventions deserve further investigation in future STI studies.

The study described here was not designed to evaluate whether there might be a change in set point viremia achieved or overall clinical benefit through transient early treatment of acute HIV infection. Larger randomized trials will be needed to determine the potential clinical and virologic benefit of therapies based on STIs. The results presented in this study suggest that the durable maintenance of low level viremia may be difficult to achieve and may also be relevant to current efforts to develop a therapeutic AIDS vaccine designed to slow down disease progression rather than prevent infection. The assessment of other interventions along with early antiretroviral therapy, in particular therapeutic vaccination, needs further testing in spite of the limited efficacy results achieved so far in treated chronic infection. In the meantime, STIs probably should be avoided outside the setting of controlled clinical trials.

References

Addo MM, Yu XG, Rathod A, Cohen D, Eldridge RL et al. Comprehensive epitope analysis of human immunodeficiency virus type 1 (HIV-1)-specific T-cell responses directed against the entire expressed HIV-1 genome demonstrate broadly directed responses, but no correlation to viral load. J Virol 2003; 77: 2081–2092

Allen TM, Kelleher AD, Zaunders J, Walker BD. STI and beyond: the prospects of boosting anti-HIV immune responses. Trends Immunol 2002; 23: 456–460

Altfeld M, Allen TM, Yu XG, Johnston MN, Agrawal D et al. HIV-1 superinfection despite broad CD8$^+$ T-cell responses containing replication of the primary virus. Nature 2002; 420: 434–439

Altfeld M, Addo MM, Shankarappa R, Lee PK, Allen TM et al. Enhanced detection of human immunodeficiency virus type 1-specific T cell responses to highly variable regions by using peptides based on autologous virus sequences. J Virol 2003; 77: 7330–7340

Autran B, Carcelain G, Li TS, Blanc C, Mathez D et al. Positive effects of combined antiretroviral therapy on CD4$^+$ T cell homeostasis and function in advanced HIV disease (see comments). Science 1997; 277: 112–116

Betts MR, Ambrozak DR, Douek DC, Bonhoeffer S, Brenchley JM et al. Analysis of total human immunodeficiency virus (HIV)-specific CD4(+) and CD8(+) T-cell responses: relationship to viral load in untreated HIV infection. J Virol 2001; 75: 11983–11991

Carcelain G, Tubiana R, Samri A, Calvez V, Delaugerre C et al. Transient mobilization of human immunodeficiency virus (HIV)-specific CD4 T-helper cells fails to control virus rebounds during intermittent antiretroviral therapy in chronic HIV type 1 infection. J Virol 2001; 75: 234–241

Cozzi Lepri A, Sabin CA, Phillips AN, Lee CA, Pezzotti P et al. The rate of CD4 decline as a determinant of progression to AIDS independent of the most recent CD4 count. The Italian Seroconversion Study. Epidemiol Infect 1998; 121: 369–376

Dean M, Carrington M, Winkler C, Huttley GA, Smith MW et al. Genetic restriction of HIV-1 infection and progression to AIDS by a deletion allele of the CKR5 structural gene. Hemophilia Growth and Development Study, Multicenter AIDS Cohort Study, Multicenter Hemophilia Cohort Study, San Francisco City Cohort, ALIVE Study. Science 1996; 273: 1856–1862

Draenert R, Verrill CL, Tang Y, Allen TM, Wurcel AG et al. Persistent recognition of autologous virus by high-avidity CD8 T cells in chronic, progressive human immunodeficiency virus type 1 infection. J Virol 2004; 78: 630–641

Fagard C, Le Braz M, Gunthard H, Hirsch HH, Egger M et al. A controlled trial of granulocyte macrophage-colony stimulating factor during interruption of HAART. AIDS 2003a; 17: 1487–1492

Fagard C, Oxenius A, Gunthard H, Garcia F, Le Braz M et al. A prospective trial of structured treatment interruptions in human immunodeficiency virus infection. Arch Intern Med 2003b; 163: 1220–1226

Finzi D, Blankson J, Siliciano JD, Margolick JB, Chadwick K et al. Latent infection of CD4$^+$ T cells provides a mechanism for lifelong persistence of HIV-1, even in patients on effective combination therapy (see comments). Nat Med 1999; 5: 512–517

Hoen B, Fournier I, Charreau I, Lacabaratz C, Burgard M et al. Structured treatment interruptions in primary HIV infection: Final results of the multicenter prospective PRIMSTOP Pilot Trial (abstract). San Francisco, USA: 11th Conference on Retroviruses and Opportunistic Infection, 2004; available under http://www.retroconference.org/2004/cd/Abstract/395.htm

Kaslow RA, Carrington M, Apple R, Park L, Munoz A et al. Influence of combinations of human major histocompatibility complex genes on the course of HIV-1 infection. Nat Med 1996; 2: 405–411

Kaufmann DE, Lichterfeld M, Altfeld M, Allen TM, Addo MM et al. Limited durability of viral control following treated acute HIV infection. PLoS Medicine 2004; 1: e36

Kinloch S, Perrin L, Hoen B, Lampe F, Phillips A et al. Evaluation of 2 Therapeutic HIV vaccination regimens in HAART-treated primary HIV infection subjects following analytical treatment interruption: QUEST PROB3005, a randomized, placebo-controlled study. San Francisco, USA: 11th Conference on Retroviruses and Opportunistic Infection, 2004; available under http://www.retroconference.org/2004/cd/Abstract/168.htm

Lafeuillade A, Poggi C, Hittinger G, Counillon E, Emilie D. Predictors of plasma human immunodeficiency virus type 1 RNA control after discontinuation of highly active antiretroviral therapy initiated at acute infection combined with structured treatment interruptions and immune-based therapies. J Infect Dis 2003; 188: 1426–1432

Lawrence J, Mayers DL, Hullsiek KH, Collins G, Abrams DI et al. Structured treatment interruption in patients with multidrug-resistant human immunodeficiency virus. N Engl J Med 2003; 349: 837–846

Lee SK, Xu Z, Lieberman J, Shankar P. The functional CD8 T cell response to HIV becomes type-specific in progressive disease. J Clin Invest 2002; 110: 1339–1347

Lichterfeld M, Yu XG, Waring MT, Mui SK, Johnston MN et al. HIV-1-specific cytotoxicity is preferentially mediated by a subset of CD8(+)T cells producing both interferon-gamma and tumor-necrosis factor-alpha. Blood 2004a; 104: 487–494

Lichterfeld M, Kaufmann DE, Yu XG, Mui SK, Addo MM et al. Loss of HIV-1-specific CD8$^+$ T cell proliferation after acute HIV-1 infection and restoration by vaccine-induced HIV-1-specific CD4$^+$ T cells. J Exp Med 2004b; 200: 701–712

Lisziewicz J, Rosenberg E, Lieberman J, Jessen H, Lopalco L et al. Control of HIV despite the discontinuation of antiretroviral therapy (letter). N Engl J Med 1999; 340: 1683–1684

Lori F, Jessen H, Lieberman J, Finzi D, Rosenberg E et al. Treatment of human immunodeficiency virus infection with hydroxyurea, didanosine, and a protease inhibitor before seroconversion is associated with normalized immune parameters and limited viral reservoir. J Infect Dis 1999; 180: 1827–1832

Lori F, Lewis MG, Xu J, Varga G, Zinn Jr DE et al. Control of SIV rebound through structured treatment interruptions during early infection. Science 2000; 290: 1591–1593

Maggiolo F, Ripamonti D, Gregis G, Quinzan G, Callegaro A et al. Effect of prolonged discontinuation of successful antiretroviral therapy on CD4 T cells: a controlled, prospective trial. AIDS 2004; 18: 439–446

Markowitz M, Jin X, Hurley A, Simon V, Ramratnam B et al. Discontinuation of antiretroviral therapy commenced early during the course of human immunodeficiency virus type 1 infection, with or without adjunctive vaccination. J Infect Dis 2002; 186: 634–643

Migueles SA, Sabbaghian MS, Shupert WL, Bettinotti MP, Marincola FM et al. HLA B*5701 is highly associated with restriction of virus replication in a subgroup of HIV-infected long term nonprogressors. Proc Natl Acad Sci USA 2000; 97: 2709–2714

Migueles SA, Laborico AC, Shupert WL, Sabbaghian MS, Rabin R et al. HIV-specific CD8$^+$ T cell proliferation is coupled to perforin expression and is maintained in nonprogressors. Nat Immunol 2002; 3: 1061–1068

Ortiz GM, Nixon DF, Trkola A, Binley J, Jin X et al. HIV-1-specific immune responses in subjects who temporarily contain virus replication after discontinuation of highly active antiretroviral therapy [see comments]. J Clin Invest 1999; 104: R13–18

Ortiz GM, Wellons M, Brancato J, Vo HT, Zinn RL et al. Structured antiretroviral treatment interruptions in chronically HIV-1-infected subjects. Proc Natl Acad Sci USA 2001; 98: 13288–13293

Oxenius A, Price DA, Gunthard HF, Dawson SJ, Fagard C et al. Stimulation of HIV-specific cellular immunity by structured treatment interruption fails to enhance viral control in chronic HIV infection. Proc Natl Acad Sci USA 2002; 99: 13747–13752

Palella Jr FJ, Delaney KM, Moorman AC, Loveless MO, Fuhrer J et al. Declining morbidity and mortality among patients with advanced human immunodeficiency virus infection. HIV Outpatient Study Investigators. N Engl J Med 1998; 338: 853–860

Richman DD. HIV chemotherapy. Nature 2001; 410: 995–1001

Rizzardi GP, Harari A, Capiluppi B, Tambussi G, Ellefsen K et al. Treatment of primary HIV-1 infection with cyclosporin A coupled with highly active antiretroviral therapy. J Clin Invest 2002; 109: 681–688

Robbins GK, Addo MM, Troung H, Rathod A, Haheeb K et al. Augmentation of HIV-1-specific T helper cell responses in chronic HIV-1 infection by therapeutic immunization. AIDS 2003; 17: 1121–1126

Rosenberg ES, Billingsley JM, Caliendo AM, Boswell SL, Sax PE et al. Vigorous HIV-1-specific CD4+ T cell responses associated with control of viremia (see comments). Science 1997; 278: 1447–1450

Rosenberg ES, Altfeld M, Poon SH, Phillips MN, Wilkes BM et al. Immune control of HIV-1 after early treatment of acute infection. Nature 2000; 407: 523–526

Tebas P, Henry K, Mondy K, Deeks S, Valdez H et al. Effect of prolonged discontinuation of successful antiretroviral therapy on CD4$^+$ T cell decline in human immunodeficiency virus-infected patients: implications for intermittent therapeutic strategies. J Infect Dis 2002; 186: 851–854

Tillmann HL, Heiken H, Knapik-Botor A, Heringlake S, Ockenga J et al. Infection with GB virus C and reduced mortality among HIV-infected patients. N Engl J Med 2001; 345: 715–724

Wherry EJ, Blattman JN, Murali-Krishna K, van der Most R, Ahmed R. Viral persistence alters CD8 T-cell immunodominance and tissue distribution and results in distinct stages of functional impairment. J Virol 2003a; 77: 4911–4927

Wherry EJ, Teichgraber V, Becker TC, Masopust D, Kaech SM et al. Lineage relationship and protective immunity of memory CD8 T cell subsets. Nat Immunol 2003b; 4: 225–234

Xiang J, Wunschmann S, Diekema DJ, Klinzman D, Patrick KD et al. Effect of coinfection with GB virus C on survival among patients with HIV infection. N Engl J Med 2001; 345: 707–714

2.4 Therapeutic Vaccination in PHI

T. P. T. Ramacciotti, D. E. Smith, S. Emery, A. D. Kelleher, D. A. Cooper

Introduction

Currently, five percent or less of those persons infected with HIV have access to treatment that effectively delays disease progression (Gotch et al., 2001; Autran et al., 2003). While the rate of new infections continues to expand disproportionately in developing regions, the percentage having access to such treatment becomes even more divergent. Moreover, there are substantial shortcomings in approaches solely reliant upon antiretroviral therapy (ART), such as toxicity, non-uniform adherence, emergence of drug resistant viral strains, cost, and delivery.

Prevention interventions based on behavioral strategies have so far met with limited success. Combined with the lack of an effective prophylactic vaccine to date, and the drawbacks of ART briefly addressed above, there is a clear need for an alternative, biological method for the prevention of disease progression in those already infected.

This chapter will examine the efforts made to date in the development of therapeutic vaccination as such a treatment strategy. This chapter covers pertinent aspects of immune system responses and summarizes results of clinical trials, comparing findings in chronic and acute infection. The various laboratory methods and standards by which candidate vaccine efficacy has been measured, as well as issues to be addressed in future, phase III and IV trials are outlined. A final section discusses the advances made and highlights the questions remaining unanswered.

The Immunology of Acute Infection

During primary HIV infection there is a rapid cascade of immunologic and virologic events. For mucosal exposure, where the majority of transmissions occur, virus is introduced into dendritic cells expressing the CD4 and the CCR5 co-receptor.

These cells then migrate to their regional lymph nodes and present antigens to resident lymphocytes (Heeney and Hahn, 2000). By approximately day 3 post-infection, the virus is circulating systemically (Fig. 2.**8**).

Plasma levels of viral replication increase exponentially and are detectable by sensitive methods, such as RNA PCR, in as few as three to five days post-infection (Wei et al., 1995; Perelson et al., 1996; Kaufmann et al., 1998; Little et al., 1999). Circulating $CD4^+$ T cells decline sharply, which may reflect their activation and pursuant infection, combined with apoptosis, concomitantly with the mounting plasma viremia and lymphoid sequestration.

Approximately 14 days post-infection, on average, the onset of clinical symptoms of acute retroviral syndrome will appear in 50–80% of individuals (Vanhems et al., 1997; Vanhems and Beaulieu, 1997; Hecht et al., 2002). The number and intensity of these symptoms are indicative of future disease progression (Vanhems et al., 1998 a; Vanhems et al., 1998 b), and often sufficient to prompt the newly infected person to seek medical care.

Following the initial viremia and CD4 decline, there is typically another inversion in which viral burden drops by log orders of magnitude, and CD4 cells rebound, though not to pre-infection levels. At approximately day 15 to 24 post-infection (Lindback et al., 2000), the individual will seroconvert, i.e., the presence of antibodies to HIV antigen will become detectable by third generation standard laboratory screening methods such as EIA as well as by Western blotting (Fig. 2.**9**).

During this period of initial infection the immune response is brisk and vigorous. Often by as early as 40 days post-infection, a rebound in CD4 cell counts and a decrease in plasma viral burden suggest that the first immune responses to the infection have been successful in at least partially controlling viral replication.

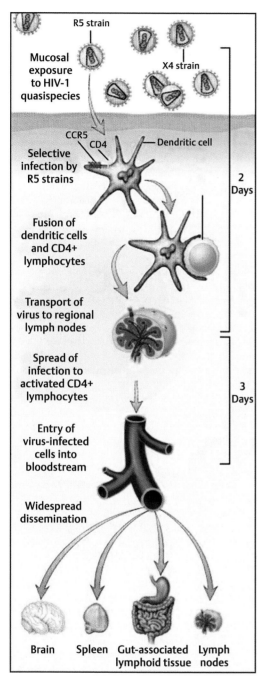

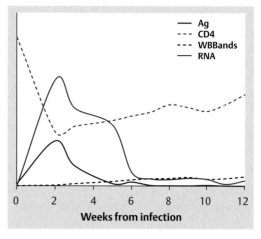

Fig. 2.9 Data from the Australian Primary HIV Infection Database: mean values in untreated patients.

However, it is at this stage that HIV infection differs from most other common viral infection models in humans. Rather than continuing to clear virus beyond the level of its initial decline, from this point onward the immune system fails to clear or even contain the infection, in all but two special populations: the long-term non-progressors and the highly-exposed seronegatives. Viral replication proceeds at levels somewhat variable between individuals, but fluctuating fairly predictably from the initial set point, a marker consistently proven to predict subsequent disease course (Lyles et al., 2000).

It is well established that HIV is rapidly adaptive to selection pressures. Even during the period immediately following transmission, the virus may revert to a form more similar to wild type in response to genetic or chemotherapeutic differences between the source and recipient environments. Several works are currently underway to more exactly characterize the extent and speed of this phenomenon (Mallal, 2004). If it can be assumed, however, that the virus remains more homogeneous in character during the first 40 to 60 days of infection than in later phases of disease, logic dictates that it is qualitative changes in the various immune responses during this narrow window of time that are responsible for the loss of containment.

One seeming failure in the initial host reaction to HIV infection is the innate component of the immune response. By virtue of its immediacy, this ancestral portion of immunity offers the host a relative grace period in most diseases, a period during which the adaptive response can be mounted. Comprised of phagocytic or proteolytic components that recognize recurring pathogens, the innate response is able to directly attack foreign antigen. As noted by Kandil et al., the innate component of the immune response to HIV infection has until now been largely unexplored, although two aspects might gainfully be investigated in greater detail. One is their suggestion that innate immunity – either instead of or in addition to adaptive response – may be responsible for the continued protective effect seen in the highly exposed seronegative population (Kandil et al., 2003). A second indication of the potential interplay of innate components in the context of HIV has been described by Gascon et al. from UCSF (Gascon et al., 2002). This group showed that, for those treatment-naïve individuals whose monocytes persistently expressed HLA-DR during primary infection, rate of loss of CD4 was greater and the response to HAART was less than in patients not expressing these monocyte activation markers. This finding contrasts with other studies of this activation marker in sepsis or post-trauma, in which increased HLA-DR expression has been shown to be consistently predictive of improved clinical outcome and survival (Hershman et al., 1990; Lekkou et al., 2004). In the context of HIV, this increased expression may simply be a consequence of immune hyperstimulation and not in itself causal or, conversely, may indicate that a stronger innate response facilitates T cell infection by increased antigen presentation.

It has been demonstrated that most neutralizing antibodies to HIV are generally weak during primary infection (Fenyo et al., 1996). Moreover, whatever response these antibodies do provide, HIV has nevertheless been shown to evade it by shifting the conformation of its envelope's glycan shield (Wei et al., 2003). It has also been suggested, however, that an antibody alone may not determine its initial neutralizing ability and that, in addition, the number or quality of professional antigen presenting cells and NK cells are a factor (Forthal et al., 2001; Wahren and Landay, 2002).

While the antibody response has been shown to be stronger later, during chronic infection, two observations seem to indicate that even this more mature and increased response is still inadequate; the first is that maternal neutralizing antibody levels do not correlate with the rate of vertical transmission; the second is that the intervening time span is sufficient for viral escape (Wei et al.,

2003). Nevertheless, at least one phase I trial exploring provision of a neutralizing antibody response using exogenous monoclonal antibodies has shown that such a response can control plasma viral load and maintain CD4/CD8 counts at least transiently (Stiegler et al., 2002). Although small, this pilot study nevertheless provides proof of the efficacy of a neutralizing antibody treatment modality.

An additional contributor to the loss of control during the acute infection period, the population of HIV-specific CD4 helper cells, which could potentially evoke and support an effector CD8 CTL response, is infected preferentially and depleted (Lederman and Douek, 2003). It has been suggested that this depletion is in part responsible for the observed decline in viral burden – because the virus has reduced the population of cells in which it can productively replicate, virion levels therefore necessarily decline.

Given the failure of these components of the immune system early on, much work has focused on the cytotoxic activity of CD8 cells, the HIV-specific CTL response. CD8 responses may be either direct (target cell lysis) or indirect (chemokine production such as RANTES, MIP-1α, and MIP-1β). Ogg et al. (1998) described a significant inverse correlation between specific CTL frequency and plasma viral load. As the latter has proven to be a reliable surrogate marker for disease progression, it would seem reasonable to assume that as CTL increases, plasma viral load decreases, and disease progression is delayed.

Parallel lines of evidence also suggest the importance of the CTL response. Simian models show that when such responses are depleted, SIV viremia remains significantly higher and disease progression is more rapid, trends which revert on reintroduction of the effector cells (Stebbings et al., 1998; Schmitz et al., 1999). Accumulating data from the highly exposed seronegative (Rowland-Jones et al., 1998 a; Rowland-Jones et al., 1998 b; Kulkarni et al., 2003) and long-term non-progressor populations (Bollinger, 1996) infer a critical, protective role for this immune response in humans.

Along this line of reasoning, many candidate HIV vaccines, in both seronegative and seropositive subjects, have used CTL response as a basis for evaluation. The trials carried out in humans up to the present are described in the next three sections of this chapter. Further discussion of CTL responses, as well as methods commonly used to assess them, will be taken up again in the penultimate portion of this chapter.

Immunization Trials in Chronically Infected Patients

Proposals for trials of HIV-1 vaccination in persons already infected with the virus, termed either therapeutic vaccination or immunotherapy, began only a few years after the isolation and identification of HIV. In the intervening years, more than 40 studies have explored the use of candidate vaccines, examining a spectrum of varying constructs, adjuvants, timing or mode of delivery applied at various disease stages.

Trials of therapeutic vaccine candidates have now been undertaken in almost 8000 human subjects. Evaluation of efficacy in the majority of these trial subjects has focused on clinical disease progression as primary endpoints, with additional or secondary endpoints measuring the effect on CD4, plasma viral load, or CTL activity.

Vaccine candidates tested to date may be classified into five major groups: a) subunits of HIV envelope; b) inactivated virus with envelope components removed; c) avian pox viruses either as single agents or in combination with envelope subunits; d) DNA constructs; and e) other HIV components or constructs (VLP, lipopeptides). These studies are summarized in Table 2.**3**.

As a class, the most extensively studied agent in the chronically infected population has been HIV envelope subunits. Collectively, these agents have been tested in more than 4000 seropositive participants, primarily in randomized, controlled trial settings. Of the envelope components, gp120 and gp160 have been the most widely studied, either as single agents, or in combination with other vaccination agents, with or without concurrent antiretroviral therapy.

Immunogen, or REMUNE, has been the next most widely tested candidate vaccine. By a series of purification and related processing steps, this inactivated virus (a strain originally of Zairian isolation) is stripped of gp120, and then emulsified in incomplete Freund's adjuvant. Evaluated most often in the asymptomatic, chronically infected populations, this agent has shown variable induction of improvement in CD4 absolute counts and percentages, and has further been tested in study populations where strains other than Clade B predominate. Across all trials this agent has been administered to > 3500 individuals.

A number of much smaller studies have used virus-like particles (VLP) or lipopeptides, either as single agents or in combination with antiretroviral therapy. While two trials evaluated the efficacy of this type of agent based on clinical progression, the primary outcomes under this approach have more typically been laboratory assessment of immunogenicity.

More recently, experiments have been undertaken using new methods in antigen delivery or induction: trials using either recombinant viral vectors, especially canarypox, DNA constructs aimed at expression of various HIV regulatory proteins such as *rev*, *nef*, and *tat*, with or without a prime-boost strategy, or delivery of inactivated virus via infected autologous dendritic cells have been described. The numbers of subjects in these studies have so far been small, and results therefore difficult to extrapolate.

Taken collectively, it may be said that results of all of these trials have been disappointing. While, as a rule, the various candidate therapies have been safe and well tolerated, none that have evaluated efficacy as measured by progression to AIDS or death have so far shown statistical significance, even when laboratory measures of T cell responses seemed promising.

Given the consistency of these negative findings, several points must be addressed: how is the disparity between laboratory and clinical response to be explained? Likewise, is the failure of therapeutic vaccination in these subjects a reflection of ineffective agents? Alternatively, are chronically infected patients the wrong study population in which to assess vaccine efficacy, regardless of whether or not their need for such a vaccine is greatest? In brief, the apparent disparity between *ex vivo* and *in vivo* results may have several causes, among which are intra-assay variation using identical methods; discordant sensitivities and specificities between different assay methods; measurement of incorrect or irrelevant surrogate markers.

The lack of clinical efficacy in this population may be a function of the degree of immune damage already incurred. Chronically infected subjects have both diminished HIV-specific CTL responses as well as demonstrated anergy to antigens and mitogens standardly used to measure immune reactivity, such as tetanus toxoid, tuberculin, and influenza. In the pre-HAART era, one early argument for the continuation of these trials, in spite of the apparent lack of success, was that no response **could** be seen in this population until lymphocytes were produced faster than they are infected, and at least a basic level of immune restoration was attained. More specifically, it was argued that the presence of replicating virus and the ongoing infection of CD4/CD8 cells compromised the efficacy

Table 2.**3**   Therapeutic vaccination studies in chronic infection

Ref	Class	Endpoints/ evaluation	Study population	N	Agent	Year Pub
	ENV					
Redfield et al., 1991		lab only	Walter Reed stage 1 – 2	30	gp160	1991
Lundholm et al., 1994		lab only	CD4 > 400	40	gp160	1994
Eron et al., 1996		clin. course and lab	CD4 > 600	573	gp120	1996
Kundu et al., 1997		lab only	CD4 > 300	76	gp160	1997
Connor et al., 1998		lab only	seroneg. converting during trial	18	gp120	1998
Kundu et al., 1998		lab only	CD4 > 500	10	gp160	1998
Leandersson et al., 1998		clin. course and lab	CD4 > 400	40	gp160	1998
Pontesilli et al., 1998		clin. course and lab	CD4 400 – 600	96	gp160	1998
Cox et al., 1999		clin. course and lab	CD4 > 400	124	gp160	1999
Goebel et al., 1999		clin. course and lab	mixed	208	gp160	1999
Ratto-Kim et al., 1999		lab only	CD4 > 400	608	gp160	1999
Sandstrom and Wahren, 1999		clin. course and lab	CD4 > 200	835	gp160	1999
Sitz et al., 1999		lab only	mixed, CD4 > 200	51	gp120 or gp160	1999
Birx et al., 2000		clin. course and lab	> 400	806	gp160	2000
DeMaria Jr et al., 2000		clin. course and lab	late stage	142	gp160	2000
Schooley et al., 2000		CD4, RNA, T cell response	CD4 50 – > 500	298	gp120	2000
Kundu-Raychaudhuri et al., 2001		T cell, CD4, stim. index	CD4 > 200	25	gp160	2001
	REMUNE					
Slade et al., 1992		CD4, DNA, p24	CD4 > 600	48	Remune	1992
Trauger et al., 1994		CD4, DTH	CD4 > 550	103	Remune	1994
Levine et al., 1996		clin. course and lab	late stage	25	Remune	1996
Churdboonchart et al., 1998		CD4, body weight, W blot	Thai, CD4 > 300	30	Remune	1998
Churdboonchart et al., 2000		CD4, CD8, weight, RNA, DTH	Thai, asympt., CD4 > 300	297	Remune	2000
Kahn et al., 2000		AIDS, death, CD4, RNA	CD4 300 – 550	2527	Remune	2000

continuation next page

Table 2.**3** Therapeutic vaccination studies in chronic infection *(continuation)*

Ref	Class	Endpoints/ evaluation	Study population	N	Agent	Year Pub
Maino et al., 2000		lab only	mixed	18	Remune	2000
Moss et al., 2000		lab only	CD4 > 400 and suppressed	11	Remune	2000
Turner et al., 2001		substudy, CD4 and virology	CD4 300 – 550	256	Remune	2001
Robbins et al., 2003		CTL, CD4	CD4 > 250, vl < 500	10	Remune	2003
Valdez et al., 2003		CD4, RNA	late stage	38	Remune	
	CP					
Engelmayer et al., 2001		lab only	mixed	9	canarypox	2001
Ratto-Kim et al., 2003		lab only	CD4 > 400	6	canarypox ± rgp160	2003
Levy et al., 2003		lab only	CD4 > 350 and suppressed	70	canarypox ± IL-2	2003
	DNA					
MacGregor et al., 1998		clin. course and lab	CD4 > 500	15	DNA	1998
Calarota et al., 1999		clin. course and lab	prev vac w/env; asymptomatic	9	DNA	1999
	OTHER					
Klein et al., 1996		lab	CD4 > 350	74	VLP	1996
Kelleher et al., 1998		clin. course and lab	CD4 > 400	61	VLP	1998
Smith et al., 2001		clin. course and lab	CD4 < 350	304	VLP	2001
Cosma et al., 2003		lab only	mixed	10	MVA nef	2003
Pinto et al., 1999; Seth et al., 2000		lab only	CD4 > 500	9	LIPOPRO-TEIN	2000
Pinto et al., 1999		lab only	CD4 > 500	8	PCLUS	1999
Sha et al., 2004		lab only	HLA B7 CD4 > 400, suppressive ART	9	C4-V3	2004
Lejeune et al., 2003		lab only	suppressive ART	12	dendritic, inactivated	2003

of vaccination. Subsequent negative results in the post-HAART era, however, suggest that this argument is false.

Autologous Vaccination and Structured Treatment Interruptions

Early results from a number of studies appear to demonstrate support for the positive immunomodulatory effects of structured treatment interruption (STI) as a therapeutic approach in primary infection (Rosenberg et al., 2000; Zaunders et al., 2003; Smith et al., 2004). In brief, this form of treatment involves viral suppression via HAART, followed by cessation of therapy for either set periods of time (typically weeks or months), or until a predetermined viral rebound is reached. Given previous findings that CTL responses are more robust when some level of viral replication is present (Ortiz et al., 2002), in theory CTL responses will be faster and stronger with each successive viral rebound following ART interruption, thus inducing essentially a self-vaccination.

Autologous vaccination may offer two additional benefits. First, each interruption allows the subjects a brief treatment respite, with expected decreased toxicities and expense. Secondly, the induced vaccination, since it is by an autologous rather than a heterologous viral strain, should allow any induced immune response to be specific for the viral strain infecting the individual subject, whereas an exogenous strain might theoretically have less specific immunogenicity. However, this latter point highlights that such specificity may also be a disadvantage and may not protect against heterologous strains. Several case reports of individuals previously well-controlled, undergoing either STI or continuous HAART regimens, have been unable to maintain such suppression upon superinfection, even when the superinfecting strains were local homologues (Altfeld et al., 2002; Jost et al., 2002).

Although this strategy has proven consistently unsuccessful in chronically infected persons (Calarote and Weiner, 2003), acutely infected patients have shown more promising early responses to this treatment modality. While the treatment interruption studies in the acute and early-infected have been small and non-randomized, a number of ongoing or soon-to-be-commenced trials (PULSE, SPARTAC, AIEDRP AI502) are investigating the utility of this treatment regimen in a systematic fashion.

Immunization Studies in Acute Infection

There are few publications on the use of therapeutic vaccinations in PHI. Because of this, discussion here will draw not only from those works in print, but also from orally presented data from recent conferences not yet in print or in press.

One of the first descriptions of therapeutic vaccination in the context of early infection was reported by Markowitz et al. (2002) from ADARC (Tab. 2.4). In a set of sixteen patients identified and commenced on HAART an average of 62 days post-onset of acute retroviral syndrome symptoms, all patients were virologically suppressed at baseline and had been treated for a mean duration of 3.2 years. Prior to voluntary cessation of treatment, eleven of the sixteen received a combination of ALVAC vCP1452 and recombinant gp160, with the remaining five subjects who were not vaccinated serving as the comparator group. Although the main outcome measures of this study – namely decline in CD4, viral rebound, and T cell proliferative responses – were similar between groups, and no correlation was found between the rate or magnitude of these markers with respect to vaccinated or control group, two observations from this study merit attention. Firstly, there appeared to be a transient period of viral suppression during the follow-up period and prior to the recommencement of HAART. Secondly, although increased CTL responses were seen during the period following treatment cessation, the investigators were not able to detect a significant correlation between these responses and the observed viral kinetics.

Along these same lines of investigation, results from three additional studies were presented early in 2004 at the 11th International Conference on Retroviruses and Opportunistic Infections (CROI) in San Francisco. All three studies reported were blinded, randomized controlled trials in acutely HIV-infected subjects.

The first study reported on at CROI, Quest or PROB3005, was quite similar in patient make-up to that reported on by Markowitz et al. Seventy-nine adult subjects on long-term suppressive HAART since primary HIV infection, were randomized on three continents to receive either placebo, vCP1452, or vCP1452 combined with inactivated, gp-120-depleted HIV, followed by discontinuation of HAART. Analysis was by intent to treat, and the primary end-point was the difference in proportions of subjects with plasma viral load ≤ 1000 copies/mL at 24 weeks post discontinuation of therapy.

Consistent with the patients from ADARC, the Quest study did not demonstrate an observable difference between vaccinated and placebo groups in plasma viral load or in CD4 decline (Kinloch et al., 2004). In contrast to the ADARC group, however, CTL response appeared to be significantly higher in the vaccinated versus the placebo group.

A second therapeutic vaccine trial in subjects with primary infection was reported on by the ANRS095 Study Group. In this trial, 43 patients with sustained virological control on HAART were assigned to either continued HAART alone or in conjunction with either IL-2, or ALVAC1433 + HIV lipopeptide 6 T. Subjects continuing to demonstrate viral control at study week 40 were eligible to discontinue HAART and were monitored for time to virologic failure as defined by plasma viral load > 50,000 at week 44 or > 10,000 at week 48. While not reaching statistical significance, the percentage of subjects remaining off HAART was higher in the IL-2 (43%) and IL-2 plus lipopeptide (49%) arms versus the HAART-only control arm (29%) (Goujard et al., 2004).

Findings from the third PHI therapeutic vaccination study (hereafter, the NCHECR study) presented at this year's CROI exemplify the converse of this observation. As in the two studies described above, all subjects were identified and treatment commenced during primary infection. During the initial safety study period, subjects received suppressive HAART and either placebo, fowlpox virus encoding *gag* and *pol* only, or fowlpox virus encoding *gag* and *pol* plus interferon-γ (IFN-γ). Twelve months after their commencement in the safety study, participants were given the opportunity to participate in an extension study. After receiving a booster (4th dose) of the same treatment as originally assigned, 25 participants ceased their antiretroviral therapy. Viral load was measured almost every week for 20 weeks. The primary endpoint for the extension study was the time-weighted mean change from the participants' baseline plasma viral load. Analysis showed that the change from baseline plasma viral load was 0.96 log10 copies/mL for patients receiving vaccine plus IFN-γ compared to 1.80 log10 for those on placebo, $p = 0.06$ (Cooper et al., 2004).

Although the observed differences in plasma viral load did not reach statistical significance, the trend is strongly suggestive of a beneficial treatment effect. However, a larger sample size, or a larger difference treatment effect between arms, or a greater follow-up time are required to reliably test the hypothesis. This finding again raises the point, however, of an apparent disparity between an observable clinical benefit in conjunction with failure to show any difference in HIV-specific CTL responses between treatment arms.

One further double-blind, randomized controlled trial in primary infection, results of which are

Table 2.**4** Completed therapeutic vaccination studies in primary infection

Ref	Popn*	Tx Duration**	Vax agent	N	Outcomes	ATI length
Markowitz et al., 2002	A & E	3 years	vCP1452 and rGP160 vs. control	16	NS: viral rebound, LPA, CD4 decline; no clinical progression	11 months
Kinloch et al., 2004	A	1.5 years	vCP1452 ± Remune vs. control	79	NS: viral rebound, LPA, CD4 decline; no clinical progression	6 months
Goujard et al., 2004	E	1 year	ALVAC1433 + LIPO-6 T vs. IL-2 vs. control	43	NS: Vax, IL-2 arms greater % off tx, less CD4 loss at wk 52	12 months
Cooper et al., 2004	A & E	1 year	Avipox-gag-pol ± IFN-γ vs. control	35	NS: lower VL rebound in vax + IFN-γ vs. vax and control (trend p = 0.06); NS: ELISpot SFU pooled vax arms vs. control p = 0.06	12 months

*   A = acute, E = early infection
**   Suppressive HAART prior to analytical treatment interruption
NS   not statistically significant

not yet published but have been briefly reviewed (Calarota and Weiner, 2003), involved the use of a DNA vaccine coding for *env/rev* plus *gag/pol*, in combination with HAART. Undertaken by MacGregor et al. at the University of Pennsylvania, the results of this trial suggest a difference in viral load, similar to those transiently seen in the ADARC study and those observed in the NCHECR study.

As a result of these promising initial findings, larger phase II and III trials are under development. Moreover, at least fifteen therapeutic vaccination trials are underway or in planning stages in Australia, Europe, and the United States, as listed in Table 2.**5**.

Concerns for Future Therapeutic Vaccination Trials

Going forward with the hypothesis that acute and early infection provide the framework in which therapeutic vaccination may best be evaluated, the following are issues that future trials will need to address, either in study design, outcomes to be measured, or other hurdles to overcome in achieving eventual licensure.

There is general consensus that an ideal therapeutic vaccine would induce multiple protective responses, including cross-reactive neutralizing antibodies, broader, stronger, and more rapid HIV-specific T cell responses, and potentially stimulated innate responses as well. No single agent evaluated to date has demonstrated significant response in all of these areas. A strategy either to employ multiple agents in combination or a novel construction simultaneously inducing several different responses is likely to have the best chance of success.

Assuming that preliminary safety profiles are acceptable, the crux of further evaluations will be efficacy, proportional to stage of evaluation. How efficacy will be measured will depend on the trial phase; however, several themes are likely to consistently apply.

For eventual licensure, candidate vaccines will need to prove utility comparable to the current standard of care. In studies with longer term follow-up, endpoints would necessarily include HIV disease progression, AIDS-defining events, and death.

In shorter term, earlier phase studies, it would be reasonable to expect that few or no such clinical events would be observed, given the brief length of infection of acutely infected trial subjects. There-

fore, proven predictors of later progression are likely to form the core of early efficacy measurement, such as plasma viral load and CD4 cell counts, in addition to any laboratory evidence of immunogenicity.

To gauge comparative performance between therapeutic vaccination and the current standard of care (such as continued ART), trials are apt to increasingly make use of analytic treatment interruptions (ATI), in which HAART is ceased and subjects are monitored in the post-intervention period in order to characterize the effects of the intervention in the absence of HAART.

In trial designs such as these, many variations upon the themes of viral and T cell function might be used as endpoints. A few of the more frequently suggested benchmarks are: effect on initial viral set point; time to start or restart of ART; number of viral blips; time to development of resistance mutations; and rates of CD4 increase or decrease.

If a candidate vaccine is found to produce a significant difference in one or more of the markers just described, discussion is likely to then revolve around several further qualities of the response; namely those of durability, magnitude, cost-benefit, and population effect. For instance, would a decrease in one-half log10 of viral load, sustained via vaccination for a one-year period be seen as sufficiently effective? For a given cost of production and schedule of administration, how does the proposed agent compare? How might the observed reduction in viral load, even of limited duration, translate into decreased rates of transmission and of new infection, likewise on transmission of resistant strains?

Laboratory Assessment of Therapeutic Vaccine Efficacy

HIV-positive individuals maintain relatively high CD8 counts and percentages throughout most of the course of their disease (Figs. 2.**10** and 2.**11**). However, while a given absolute cell count may be necessary (as seen with CD4 cells), numbers alone do not reflect adequate immune control, hence the emphasis in recent years on the qualitative responses of cytotoxic T lymphocytes. In order to measure these T cell responses, a small number of assays are routinely used. Sun et al. have provided a detailed, quantitative comparison of these methods (Sun et al., 2003). The essential features of each are briefly described here.

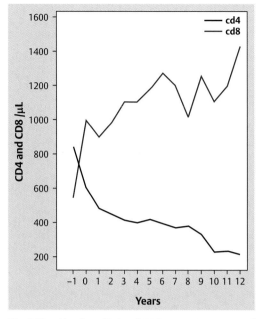

Fig. 2.**10**   Absolute CD4 and CD8 counts in untreated patients, by time from infection.

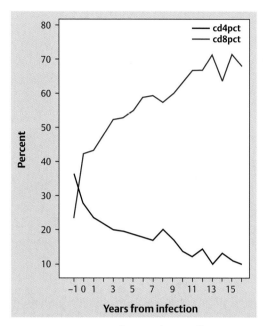

Fig. 2.**11**   Percentage of CD4 and CD8 cells in untreated patients, by time from infection.

The lymphoproliferative assay (LPA) essentially measures the degree to which CD4 cells clonally expand in response to a given antigenic or mitogenic stimulus. A stimulation index based on this assay describes the ratio of expansion in cells exposed to the antigen to those cells which were not exposed to the antigen. While a minority of these CD4 cells may have direct cytotoxic effects of their own, the majority of CTL is carried out by CD8 lymphocytes; therefore, the LPA provides some measure of the potential for mediated cell lysis, but no direct measure of these processes. Most studies to date have used a stimulation index of five-fold greater than control as a meaningful response.

In contrast, the chromium release assay directly measures target cell lysis by CTL. This assay detects the amount of chromium released by target cells upon exposure to T lymphocytes and subsequent destruction. The chromium is absorbed by the target cells during incubation prior to addition of CTL. A range of ± ten percent is typical for this assay, based on the observed release of free chromium by the target cells not exposed to CTL.

Two assays increasingly used to determine T cell effector activity are the ELISPOT and intracellular cytokine staining (ICS) methods. ELISPOT is an ELISA format assay, primarily used for measurement of IFN-γ production. In this assay, CTL effec-

tor cells are quantified by the number of spots formed on the assay plate, indicating where these cells have released cytokine.

ICS is also a method for measurement of cytokine production, making use of antigen to induce the cytokine production combined with antibodies to cell surface markers and the intracellularly-produced cytokine(s) of interest, together with an intermediate step to inhibit extracellular release of the produced cytokines. The final step is then detection of the bound antibody to the cytokine and surface marker combinations of interest, by multicolor flow cytometry.

Tetramer staining involves the use of soluble, HLA class I multimers, and enumerates the number of T cells specific for a particular epitope. These multimers are peptide complexes specific for the T cell receptors (TCRs) of the lymphocytes being evaluated. The multimers are produced to bind with high avidity to the TCR and are labeled for subsequent detection by flow cytometry.

It should be noted that this newer method, while superior in sensitivity, is a marker of cell phenotype rather than function. Thus, while it provides an approximation of markers for *potential* immune response (such as antigen specificity, CD markers of effector versus memory, cytokine production, etc.), no assay based on antigen-specific cell numbers or

Table 2.**5**   Therapeutic vaccination trials underway

Study Number	Status	Agent	Site(s)	N
0900-397	Open	VCP1452 + IL-2	Cornell	92
AACTG 5130	Open	AUTOLOG DC VCP1452	AACTG	30
AACTG 5187	Open	PLASMID DNA	AACTG	20
AI-04-006	Open	VCP1452 + GP160	ADARC	12
AI43664-04	Open	AUTOLOG DC A2 PEPTIDE	UPITT	18
AI44628	Open	Dendritic cells pulsed with HIV antigens	MGH	10
GTU-MultiHIV	Open	NNV-Nef	FITBIOTECH	16
ACTG A5197	Phase II, in devel.	MRK Ad5 HIV-1 Gag vaccine	AACTG	120
AACTG 5024	Recruited, ongoing	HAART ± ALVAC ± IL-2	AACTG	76
AACTG 5068	Recruited, ongoing	ALVAC ± ATI	AACTG	97
EP HIV-1090	Recruited, ongoing	MULTI-EPITOPE DNA	UCHSC	40

production of a particular cytokine predicts the level of viral control induced by CD8 T cells.

A recurring theme in therapeutic vaccination studies so far has been the apparent discrepancy between a significant CTL response – at least as measured by current methods and markers – and clinical outcome. Despite initial evidence of an inverse correlation between CTL and viral load, subsequent studies have failed to reproduce or have contradicted these findings (Brander and Riviere, 2002; Lederman et al., 2003). Or, in studies where clinical benefit has been suggested, a significant immune response has not been observed.

There are at least two possible solutions to this puzzle, potentially overlapping. Either the technique is at fault, in that the "correct" biological factors are under evaluation, but measured imprecisely, or inconsistently, or inadequately, so that clinically meaningful relationships exist, but are not predictably detected. Or, the methods are technically and methodologically correct, but the measurements are of limited value in this context because the wrong aspects of CTL or other immune responses are being examined.

In summary, we now have several sensitive methods with which to describe certain aspects of the CTL function. So far, little consistent correlation has been observed between measured laboratory immunogenicity and clinical course. As vaccination trials progress to later phases in vaccine development, efficacy increasingly becomes the standard by which such trials are measured. Determination of what are the markers of cell mediated immunity that reliably predict disease progression

and rate, and how to measure such markers by high throughput, automated, and reproducible methods are issues of key importance still to be resolved.

Discussion

The randomized trials conducted to date have predominantly been among chronically infected subjects. Few would argue that this is the population in greatest need of an effective therapy. While generally well-tolerated, none of the vaccines tested in this group have thus far proven effective in slowing disease progression. The lack of response in trials on these subjects may be difficult to interpret, not only because of the demonstrated immunologic anergy in the test persons, but also because of the heterogeneity within the group with regard to time from infection and other cofactors in the rate of disease progression.

Because the number of trials in acute infection have been quite small up until now, it is difficult to speculate on outcomes of future investigations. However, the level of interest in pursuing studies in this somewhat more homogeneous group is increasing. There are at least four times as many PHI vaccination trials now underway or in development than have previously been conducted in the time since HIV was first isolated. Although attention is likely to further concentrate in this area and potentially provide proof of principle, the logistics of identifying acutely infected patients may preclude widespread applicability.

There is ample evidence from other viral models that therapeutic vaccination can successfully contain disease, particularly when administered acutely. Rabies and hepatitis B are two prominent examples, and preliminary data indicate that human papilloma and herpes simplex viruses may also respond to this method of treatment.

Evidence from these other viral models and recent results in acutely infected subjects indicate that therapeutic vaccination, as a mode for the treatment of HIV-1 infection, remains a worthy target of exploration and investigation. In comparison with currently available antiretroviral therapy, such a vaccine may reasonably be expected to be better tolerated and offer enormous economic and logistic advantages. A therapeutic vaccine even if only partially effective – a premise examined ever more frequently in current epidemiological models – would confer meaningful reductions in transmissibility and rate of disease spread, conferring profound benefit at both the individual and population levels, and thereby serve to reduce the toll of this exacting disease.

References

Altfeld M, Allen TM, Yu XG, Johnston MN, Agrawal D, Korber BT, Montefiori DC, O'Connor DH, Davis BT, Lee PK, Maier EL, Harlow J, Goulder PJ, Brander C, Rosenberg ES, Walker BD. HIV-1 superinfection despite broad CD8⁺ T-cell responses containing replication of the primary virus (see comment). Nature 2002; 420: 434–439

Autran B, Debre P, Walker B, Katlama C. Therapeutic vaccines against HIV need international partnerships. Nat Rev Immunol 2003; 3: 503–508

Birx DL, Loomis-Price LD, Aronson N, Brundage J, Davis C, Deyton L, Garner R, Gordin F, Henry D, Holloway W, Kerkering T, Luskin-Hawk R, McNeil J, Michael N, Foster Pierce P, Poretz D, Ratto-Kim S, Renzullo P, Ruiz N, Sitz K, Smith G, Tacket C, Thompson M, Tramont E, Yangco B, Yarrish R, Redfield RR. Efficacy testing of recombinant human immunodeficiency virus (HIV) gp160 as a therapeutic vaccine in early-stage HIV-1-infected volunteers. rgp160 phase II vaccine investigators. J Infect Dis 2000; 181: 881–889

Bollinger RC. Cellular immune responses to HIV-1. AIDS 1996; 10: S85–96

Brander C, Riviere Y. Early and late cytotoxic T lymphocyte responses in HIV infection. AIDS 2002; 16 (Suppl 4): S97–103

Calarota SA, Weiner DB. Present status of human HIV vaccine development. AIDS 2003; 17 (Suppl 4): S73–84

Calarota SA, Leandersson AC, Bratt G, Hinkula J, Klinman DM, Weinhold KJ, Sandstrom E, Wahren B. Immune responses in asymptomatic HIV-1-infected patients after HIV-DNA immunization followed by highly active antiretroviral treatment. J Immunol 1999; 163: 2330–2338

Churdboonchart V, Moss RB, Sirawaraporn W, Smutharaks B, Sutthent R, Jensen FC, Vacharak P, Grimes J, Theofan G, Carlo DJ. Effect of HIV-specific immune-based therapy in subjects infected with HIV-1 subtype E in Thailand. AIDS 1998; 12: 1521–1527

Churdboonchart V, Sakondhavat C, Kulpradist S, Na Ayudthya BI, Chandeying V, Rugpao S, Boonshuyar C, Sukeepaisarncharoen W, Sirawaraporn W, Carlo DJ, Moss R. A double-blind, adjuvant-controlled trial of human immunodeficiency virus type 1 (HIV-1) immunogen (Remune) monotherapy in asymptomatic, HIV-1-infected Thai subjects with CD4-cell counts of > 300 (see comment; an erratum appears in Clin Diagn Lab Immunol 2001; 8: 1295). Clin Diagn Lab Immunol 2000; 7: 728–733

Connor RI, Korber BT, Graham BS, Hahn BH, Ho DD, Walker BD, Neumann AU, Vermund SH, Mestecky J, Jackson S, Fenamore E, Cao Y, Gao F, Kalams S, Kunstman KJ, McDonald D, McWilliams N, Trkola A, Moore JP, Wolinsky SM. Immunological and virological analyses of persons infected by human immunodeficiency virus type 1 while participating in trials of recombinant gp120 subunit vaccines. J Virol 1998; 72: 1552–1576

Cooper D, Workman C et al. Randomized, placebo-controlled, phase1/2a evaluation of the safety, biological activity and antiretroviral properties of an avipox virus vaccine expressing HIV gag-pol and interferon-gamma in HIV-1 infected subjects. San Francisco: 11th Conference on Retroviruses and Opportunistic Infections, 2004

Cosma A, Nagaraj R, Buhler S, Hinkula J, Busch DH, Sutter G, Goebel FD, Erfle V. Therapeutic vaccination with MVA-HIV-1 nef elicits Nef-specific T-helper cell responses in chronically HIV-1 infected individuals. Vaccine 2003; 22: 21–29

Cox JH, Garner RP, Redfield RR, Aronson NE, Davis C, Ruiz N, Birx DL. Antibody-dependent cellular cytotoxicity in HIV type 1-infected patients receiving VaxSyn, a recombinant gp160 envelope vaccine. AIDS Res Hum Retroviruses 1999; 15: 847–854

DeMaria Jr A, Kunches L, Mayer K et al. Immune responses to a recombinant human immunodeficiency virus type 1 (HIV) gp160 vaccine among adults with advanced HIV infection. J Hum Virol 2000; 3: 182–192

Engelmayer J, Larsson M, Lee A et al. Mature dendritic cells infected with canarypox virus elicit strong anti-human immunodeficiency virus CD8⁺ and CD4⁺ T-cell responses from chronically infected individuals. J Virol 2001; 75: 2142–2153

Eron Jr JJ, Ashby MA, Giordano MF, Chernow M, Reiter WM, Deeks SG, Lavelle JP, Conant MA, Yangco BG, Pate PG, Torres RA, Mitsuyasu RT, Twaddell T. Randomised trial of MNrgp120 HIV-1 vaccine in symptomless HIV-1 infection (see comment). Lancet 1996; 348: 1547–1551

Fenyo EM, Albert J, McKeating J. The role of the humoral immune response in HIV infection. AIDS 1996; 10 (Suppl A): S97–106

Forthal DN, Landucci G, Daar ES. Antibody From Patients with Acute HIV-1 Infection Inhibits Primary Strains of HIV-1 in the Presence of Natural Killer Effector Cells. Philadelphia, PA: AIDS Vaccine, 2001

Gascon RL, Narvaez AB, Zhang R, Kahn JO, Hecht FM, Herndier BG, McGrath MS. Increased HLA-DR expression on peripheral blood monocytes in subsets of subjects with primary HIV infection is associated with elevated CD4 T-cell apoptosis and CD4 T-cell depletion. J Acquir Immune Defic Syndr 2002; 30: 146–153

Goebel FD, Mannhalter JW, Belshe RB, Eibl MM, Grob PJ, de Gruttola V, Griffiths PD, Erfle V, Kunschak M, Engl W. Recombinant gp160 as a therapeutic vaccine for HIV-infection: results of a large randomized, controlled trial. European Multinational IMMUNO AIDS Vaccine Study Group. AIDS 1999; 13: 1461–1468

Gotch FM, Imami N, Hardy G. Candidate vaccines for immunotherapy in HIV. HIV Medicine 2001; 2: 260–265

Goujard C, Marcellin F et al. HIV immune and virological responses following the administration of IL-2 either alone or combined to ALVAC-HIV 1433 and HIV lipopeptides in patients treated early with HAART during primary infection: the ANRS 095 Randomized Study. San Francisco: 11th Conference on Retroviruses and Opportunistic Infections, 2004

Hecht FM, Busch MP, Rawal B, Webb M, Rosenberg E, Swanson M, Chesney M, Anderson J, Levy J, Kahn JO. Use of laboratory tests and clinical symptoms for identification of primary HIV infection. AIDS 2002; 16: 1119–1129

Heeney JL, Hahn BH. Vaccines and immunology: elucidating immunity to HIV-1 and current prospects for AIDS vaccine development. AIDS 2000; 14 (Suppl 3): S125–127

Hershman MJ, Cheadle WG, Wellhausen SR, Davidson PF, Polk Jr HC. Monocyte HLA-DR antigen expression characterizes clinical outcome in the trauma patient. Br J Surg 1990; 77: 204–207

Jost S, Bernard MC, Kaiser L, Yerly S, Hirschel B, Samri A, Autran B, Goh LE, Perrin L. A patient with HIV-1 superinfection (see comment). N Engl J Med 2002; 347: 731–736

Kahn JO, Walker BD. Acute human immunodeficiency virus type 1 infection. N Engl J Med 1998; 339: 33–39

Kahn JO, Cherng DW, Mayer K, Murray H, Lagakos S. Evaluation of HIV-1 immunogen, an immunologic modifier, administered to patients infected with HIV having 300 to 549×10(6)/L CD4 cell counts: A randomized controlled trial (see comment; an erratum appears in JAMA 2001; 285: 2197). JAMA 2000; 284: 2193–2202

Kandil H, Stebbing J et al. Innate and adaptive immunological insights into HIV pathogenesis. Int J STD & AIDS 2003; 14: 652–655

Kaufmann GR, Cunningham P, Kelleher AD, Zaunders J, Carr A, Vizzard J, Law M, Cooper DA. Patterns of viral dynamics during primary human immunodeficiency virus type 1 infection. The Sydney Primary HIV Infection Study Group. J Infect Dis 1998; 178: 1812–1815

Kelleher AD, Roggensack M, Jaramillo AB, Smith DE, Walker A, Gow I, McMurchie M, Harris J, Patou G, Cooper DA. Safety and immunogenicity of a candidate therapeutic vaccine, p24 virus-like particle, combined with zidovudine, in asymptomatic subjects. Community HIV Research Network Investigators. AIDS 1998; 12: 175–182

Kinloch S, Perrin L et al. Evaluation of 2 therapeutic HIV vaccination regimens in HAART-treated primary HIV infection subjects following analytical treatment interruption: QUEST PROB3005, a randomized, placebo-controlled study. San Francisco: 11th Conference on Retroviruses and Opportunistic Infections, 2004

Klein MR, Veenstra J, Holwerda AM et al. Gag-specific immune responses after immunization with p17/p24:Ty virus-like particles in HIV type 1-seropositive individuals. AIDS Res Hum Retroviruses 1996; 13: 393–399

Kulkarni PS, Butera ST, Duerr AC. Resistance to HIV-1 infection: lessons learned from studies of highly exposed persistently seronegative (HEPS) individuals. AIDS Rev 2003; 5: 87–103

Kundu SK, Katzenstein D, Valentine FT, Spino C, Efron B, Merigan TC. Effect of therapeutic immunization with recombinant gp160 HIV-1 vaccine on HIV-1 proviral DNA and plasma RNA: relationship to cellular immune responses. J Acquir Immune Defic Syndr Hum Retrovirol 1997; 15: 269–274

Kundu SK, Dupuis M, Sette A, Celis E, Dorner F, Eibl M, Merigan TC. Role of preimmunization virus sequences in cellular immunity in HIV-infected patients during HIV type 1 MN recombinant gp160 immunization. AIDS Res Hum Retroviruses 1998; 14: 1669–1678

Kundu-Raychaudhuri S, Sevin A, Kilgo P, Nokta M, Pollard RB, Merigan TC. Effect of therapeutic immunization with HIV type 1 recombinant glycoprotein 160 ImmunoAG vaccine in HIV-infected individuals with CD4+ T cell counts of > or = 500 and 200–400/mm³ (AIDS Clinical Trials Group Study 246/946). AIDS Res Hum Retroviruses 2001; 17: 1371–1378

Leandersson AC, Bratt G, Hinkula J, Gilljam G, Cochaux P, Samson M, Sandstrom E, Wahren B. Induction of specific T-cell responses in HIV infection. AIDS 1998; 12: 157–166

Lederman MM, Douek DC. Sometimes help may not be enough (comment). AIDS 2003; 17: 1249–1251

Lejeune M, García F, Climent N, Gil C, Alcamí J, Morente V, Alós L, Libois A, Fumero E, Florence E, Pereira A, Caballero M, Cruceta A, Castro P, Miró JM, Plana M, Gatell JM, Gallart T. Therapeutic vaccination using autologous monocyte-derived dendritic cells (MD-

DC) loaded with inactivated autologous virus in patients with chronic HIV infection and nadir of CD4 T cells above 400. Paris: The 2nd IAS Conference on HIV Pathogenesis and Treatment, 2003

Lekkou A, Karakantza M, Mouzaki A, Kalfarentzos F, Gogos CA. Cytokine production and monocyte HLA-DR expression as predictors of outcome for patients with community-acquired severe infections. Clin Diagn Lab Immunol 2004; 11: 161 – 167

Levine A, Groshen S, Allen J et al. Initial studies on active immunization of HIV-infected subjects using a gp120-depleted HIV-1 immunogen: long-term follow-up. JAIDS 1996; 11: 351 – 363

Levy Y, Gahery-Segard H et al. Immunological and virological efficacy of ALVAC-HIV 1433 and HIV lipopeptides (Lipo-6 T) combined with SC IL-2 in chronically HIV-infected patients: results of the ANRS 093 randomized study. Boston: 10th Conference on Retroviruses and Opportunistic Infections, 2003

Lindback S, Thorstensson R, Karlsson AC, von Sydow M, Flamholc L, Blaxhult A, Sonnerborg A, Biberfeld G, Gaines H. Diagnosis of primary HIV-1 infection and duration of follow-up after HIV exposure. Karolinska Institute Primary HIV Infection Study Group. AIDS 2000; 14: 2333 – 2339

Little SJ, McLean AR, Spina CA, Richman DD, Havlir DV. Viral dynamics of acute HIV-1 infection. J Exp Med 1999; 190: 841 – 850

Lundholm P, Wahren M, Sandstrom E, Volvovitz F, Wahren B. Autoreactivity in HIV-infected individuals does not increase during vaccination with envelope rgp160. Immunol Lett 1994; 41: 147 – 153

Lyles RH, Munoz A, Yamashita TE, Bazmi H, Detels R, Rinaldo CR, Margolick JB, Phair JP, Mellors JW. Natural history of human immunodeficiency virus type 1 viremia after seroconversion and proximal to AIDS in a large cohort of homosexual men. Multicenter AIDS Cohort Study. J Infect Dis 2000; 181: 872 – 880

MacGregor RR, Boyer JD, Ugen KE, Lacy KE, Gluckman SJ, Bagarazzi ML, Chattergoon MA, Baine Y, Higgins TJ, Ciccarelli RB, Coney LR, Ginsberg RS, Weiner DB. First human trial of a DNA-based vaccine for treatment of human immunodeficiency virus type 1 infection: safety and host response (see comment). J Infect Dis 1998; 178: 92 – 100

Maino VC, Suni MA, Wormsley SB, Carlo DJ, Wallace MR, Moss RB. Enhancement of HIV type 1 antigen-specific CD4$^+$ T cell memory in subjects with chronic HIV type 1 infection receiving an HIV type 1 immunogen (erratum appears in AIDS Res Hum Retroviruses 2000; 16: 2065 – 2066). AIDS Res Hum Retroviruses 2000; 16: 539 – 547

Mallal S. HLA imprinting: implications for selection of vaccine immunogens. San Francisco: 11th Conference on Retroviruses and Opportunistic Infections, 2004

Markowitz M, Jin X, Hurley A, Simon V, Ramratnam B, Louie M, Deschenes GR, Ramanathan Jr M, Barsoum S, Vanderhoeven J, He T, Chung C, Murray J, Perelson AS, Zhang L, Ho DD. Discontinuation of antiretroviral therapy commenced early during the course of human immunodeficiency virus type 1 infection, with or without adjunctive vaccination. J Infect Dis 2002; 186: 634 – 643

Moss RB, Giermakowska W, Wallace MR, Savary J, Jensen F, Carlo DJ. T-helper-cell proliferative responses to whole-killed human immunodeficiency virus type 1 (HIV-1) and p24 antigens of different clades in HIV-1-infected subjects vaccinated with HIV-1 immunogen (Remune). Clin Diagn Lab Immunol 2000; 7: 724 – 727

Ogg GS, Jin X, Bonhoeffer S, Dunbar PR, Nowak MA, Monard S, Segal JP, Cao Y, Rowland-Jones SL, Cerundolo V, Hurley A, Markowitz M, Ho DD, Nixon DF, McMichael AJ. Quantitation of HIV-1-specific cytotoxic T lymphocytes and plasma load of viral RNA. Science 1998; 279: 2103 – 2106

Ortiz GM, Hu J, Goldwitz JA, Chandwani R, Larsson M, Bhardwaj N, Bonhoeffer S, Ramratnam B, Zhang L, Markowitz MM, Nixon DF. Residual viral replication during antiretroviral therapy boosts human immunodeficiency virus type 1-specific CD8$^+$ T-cell responses in subjects treated early after infection. J Virol 2002; 76: 411 – 415

Perelson AS, Neumann AU, Markowitz M, Leonard JM, Ho DD. HIV-1 dynamics *in vivo*: virion clearance rate, infected cell life-span, and viral generation time. Science 1996; 271: 1582 – 1586

Pinto LA, Berzofsky JA, Fowke KR, Little RF, Merced-Galindez F, Humphrey R, Ahlers J, Dunlop N, Cohen RB, Steinberg SM, Nara P, Shearer GM, Yarchoan R. HIV-specific immunity following immunization with HIV synthetic envelope peptides in asymptomatic HIV-infected patients. AIDS 1999; 13: 2003 – 2012

Pontesilli O, Guerra EC, Ammassari A, Tomino C, Carlesimo M, Antinori A, Tamburrini E, Prozzo A, Seeber AC, Vella S, Ortona L, Aiuti F. Phase II controlled trial of post-exposure immunization with recombinant gp160 versus antiretroviral therapy in asymptomatic HIV-1-infected adults. VaxSyn Protocol Team. AIDS 1998; 12: 473 – 480

Ratto-Kim S, Sitz KV, Garner RP, Kim JH, Davis C, Aronson N, Ruiz N, Tencer K, Redfield RR, Birx DL. Repeated immunization with recombinant gp160 human immunodeficiency virus (HIV) envelope protein in early HIV-1 infection: evaluation of the T cell proliferative response. J Infect Dis 1999; 179: 337 – 344

Ratto-Kim S, Loomis-Price LD, Aronson N, Grimes J, Hill C, Williams C, El Habib R, Birx DL, Kim JH. Comparison between env-specific T-cell epitopic responses in HIV-1-uninfected adults immunized with combination of ALVAC-HIV(vCP205) plus or minus rgp160 MN/LAI-2 and HIV-1-infected adults. J Acquir Immune Defic Syndr 2003; 32: 9 – 17

Redfield RR, Birx DL, Ketter N, Tramont E, Polonis V, Davis C, Brundage JF, Smith G, Johnson S, Fowler A et al. A phase I evaluation of the safety and immunogenicity of vaccination with recombinant gp160 in patients with early human immunodeficiency virus infection. Military Medical Consortium for Applied

Retroviral Research (see comment). N Engl J Med 1991; 324: 1677–1684

Robbins GK, Addo MM, Troung H, Rathod A, Habeeb K, Davis B, Heller H, Basgoz N, Walker BD, Rosenberg ES. Augmentation of HIV-1-specific T helper cell responses in chronic HIV-1 infection by therapeutic immunization (see comment). AIDS 2003; 17: 1121–1126

Rosenberg ES, Altfeld M, Poon SH, Phillips MN, Wilkes BM, Eldridge RL, Robbins GK, D'Aquila RT, Goulder PJ, Walker BD. Immune control of HIV-1 after early treatment of acute infection. Nature 2000; 407: 523–526

Rowland-Jones S, Dong T, Krausa P, Sutton J, Newell H, Ariyoshi K, Gotch F, Sabally S, Corrah T, Kimani J, MacDonald K, Plummer F, Ndinya-Achola J, Whittle H, McMichael A. The role of cytotoxic T-cells in HIV infection. Dev Biol Stand 1998a; 92: 209–214

Rowland-Jones SL, Dong T, Fowke KR, Kimani J, Krausa P, Newell H, Blanchard T, Ariyoshi K, Oyugi J, Ngugi E, Bwayo J, MacDonald KS, McMichael AJ, Plummer FA. Cytotoxic T cell responses to multiple conserved HIV epitopes in HIV-resistant prostitutes in Nairobi (see comment). J Clin Invest 1998b; 102: 1758–1765

Sandstrom E, Wahren B. Therapeutic immunisation with recombinant gp160 in HIV-1 infection: a randomised double-blind placebo-controlled trial. Nordic VAC-04 Study Group (see comment). Lancet 1999; 353: 1735–1742

Schmitz JE, Kuroda MJ, Santra S, Sasseville VG, Simon MA, Lifton MA, Racz P, Tenner-Racz K, Dalesandro M, Scallon BJ, Ghrayeb J, Forman MA, Montefiori DC, Rieber EP, Letvin NL, Reimann KA. Control of viremia in simian immunodeficiency virus infection by CD8+ lymphocytes. Science 1999; 283: 857–860

Schooley RT, Spino C, Kuritzkes D, Walker BD, Valentine FA, Hirsch MS, Cooney E, Friedland G, Kundu S, Merigan Jr TC, McElrath MJ, Collier A, Plaeger S, Mitsuyasu R, Kahn J, Haslett P, Uherova P, deGruttola V, Chiu S, Zhang B, Jones G, Bell D, Ketter N, Twadell T, Chernoff D, Rosandich M. Two double-blinded, randomized, comparative trials of 4 human immunodeficiency virus type 1 (HIV-1) envelope vaccines in HIV-1-infected individuals across a spectrum of disease severity: AIDS Clinical Trials Groups 209 and 214. J Infect Dis 2000; 182: 1357–1364

Seth A, Yasutomi Y, Jacoby H, Callery JC, Kaminsky SM, Koff WC, Nixon DF, Letvin NL. Evaluation of a lipopeptide immunogen as a therapeutic in HIV type 1-seropositive individuals. AIDS Res Hum Retroviruses 2000; 16: 337–343

Sha B, Onorato M et al. Safety and immunogenicity of a polyvalent peptide C4-V3 HIV vaccine in conjunction with IL-12. AIDS 2004; 18: 1203–1216

Sitz KV, Ratto-Kim S, Hodgkins AS, Robb ML, Birx DL. Proliferative responses to human immunodeficiency virus type 1 (HIV-1) gp120 peptides in HIV-1-infected individuals immunized with HIV-1 rgp120 or rgp160 compared with nonimmunized and uninfected controls. J Infect Dis 1999; 179: 817–824

Slade H, Turner J, Abrams C, Carlo D, Salk J. Immunotherapy of HIV-seropositive patients: preliminary report on a dose-ranging study. AIDS Res Hum Retroviruses 1992; 8: 1329–1331

Smith D, Gow I, Colebunders R, Weller I, Tchamouroff S, Weber J, Boag F, Hales G, Adams S, Patou G, Cooper DA. Therapeutic vaccination (p24-VLP) of patients with advanced HIV-1 infection in the pre-HAART era does not alter CD4 cell decline. HIV Med 2001; 2: 272–275

Smith D, Grey P et al. Virological and immunological predictors of time to initial viral suppression and viral rebound in a randomised trial of combination therapy in primary HIV infection followed by treatment interruption. San Francisco: 11th Conference on Retroviruses and Opportunistic Infections, 2004

Stebbings R, Stott J, Almond N, Hull R, Lines J, Silvera P, Sangster R, Corcoran T, Rose J, Cobbold S, Gotch F, McMichael A, Walker B. Mechanisms of protection induced by attenuated simian immunodeficiency virus. II. Lymphocyte depletion does not abrogate protection (see comment). AIDS Res Hum Retroviruses 1998; 14: 1187–1198

Stiegler G, Armbruster C, Vcelar B, Stoiber H, Kunert R, Michael NL, Jagodzinski LL, Ammann C, Jager W, Jacobson J, Vetter N, Katinger H. Antiviral activity of the neutralizing antibodies 2F5 and 2G12 in asymptomatic HIV-1-infected humans: a phase I evaluation. AIDS 2002; 16: 2019–2025

Sun Y, Iglesias E, Samri A, Kamkamidze G, Decoville T, Carcelain G, Autran B. A systematic comparison of methods to measure HIV-1 specific CD8 T cells. J Immunol Meth 2003; 272: 23–34

Trauger RJ, Ferre F, Daigle AE, Jensen FC, Moss RB, Mueller SH, Richieri SP, Slade HB, Carlo DJ. Effect of immunization with inactivated gp120-depleted human immunodeficiency virus type 1 (HIV-1) immunogen on HIV-1 immunity, viral DNA, and percentage of CD4 cells. J Infect Dis 1994; 169: 1256–1264

Turner JL, Kostman JR, Aquino A, Wright D, Szabo S, Bidwell R, Goodgame J, Daigle A, Kelley E, Jensen F, Duffy C, Carlo D, Moss RB. The effects of an HIV-1 immunogen (Remune) on viral load, CD4 cell counts and HIV-specific immunity in a double-blind, randomized, adjuvant-controlled subset study in HIV infected subjects regardless of concomitant antiviral drugs (see comment). HIV Med 2001; 2: 68–77

Valdez H, Mitsuyasu R, Landay A, Sevin AD, Chan ES, Spritzler J, Kalams SA, Pollard RB, Fahey J, Fox L, Namkung A, Estep S, Moss R, Sahner D, Lederman MM. Interleukin-2 increases CD4+ lymphocyte numbers but does not enhance responses to immunization: results of A5046 s. J Infect Dis 2003; 187: 320–325

Vanhems P, Beaulieu R. Primary infection by type 1 human immunodeficiency virus: diagnosis and prognosis. Postgrad Med J 1997; 73: 403–408

Vanhems P, Allard R, Cooper DA, Perrin L, Vizzard J, Hirschel B, Kinloch-de Loes S, Carr A, Lambert J. Acute human immunodeficiency virus type 1 disease as a mononucleosis-like illness: is the diagnosis too restrictive? (Erratum appears in Clin Infect Dis 1997; 25: 352). Clin Infect Dis 1997; 24: 965–970

Vanhems P, Lambert J, Cooper DA, Perrin L, Carr A, Hirschel B, Vizzard J, Kinloch-de Loes S, Allard R. Severity and prognosis of acute human immunodeficiency virus type 1 illness: a dose-response relationship. Clin Infect Dis 1998 a; 26: 323–329

Vanhems P, Lecomte C, Fabry J. Primary HIV-1 infection: diagnosis and prognostic impact. AIDS Patient Care & Stds 1998 b; 12: 751–758

Wahren B, Landay A. HIV immunology better understood and vaccination attempts started. AIDS 2002; 16 (Suppl 4): S85–88

Wei X, Ghosh SK, Taylor ME, Johnson VA, Emini EA, Deutsch P, Lifson JD, Bonhoeffer S, Nowak MA, Hahn BH et al. Viral dynamics in human immunodeficiency virus type 1 infection (see comment). Nature 1995; 373: 117–122

Wei X, Decker JM, Wang S, Hui H, Kappes JC, Wu X, Salazar-Gonzalez JF, Salazar MG, Kilby JM, Saag MS, Komarova NL, Nowak MA, Hahn BH, Kwong PD, Shaw GM. Antibody neutralization and escape by HIV-1. Nature 2003; 422: 307–312

Zaunders J, Munier M et al. T-cell subset perturbations during the first interruption phase of subjects treated during primary HIV infection: activation and CCR5 expression correlate with viral load. Boston: 10th Conference on Retroviruses and Opportunistic Infections, 2003

3 Clinical Epidemiology and Management

3.1 Drug Resistance and Transmission of Resistance

E. C. Bowles, C. A. B. Boucher

Abbreviations and Definitions

Fidelity
accuracy in transcription

Fitness
viral replication capacity in a given environment

Genetic barrier
the number of mutations a virus needs to acquire in order to confer resistance to a certain drug

Genotype
nucleotide sequence

HAART
highly active antiretroviral therapy

Phenotype
the way the nucleotide sequence is expressed in properties of the virus, e.g. susceptibility to drugs

Primary (resistance) mutation
a primary mutation alone confers resistance to a particular drug

Primary resistance
a patient is resistant to a drug without ever having been exposed to the drug; he has been infected with a resistant virus

Resistance
diminished susceptibility of the virus to an antiretroviral drug

Secondary (resistance) mutation
this mutation compensates for the reduced fitness of the virus in the presence of the primary mutation

Introduction

Worldwide increasing numbers of HIV-infected people are gaining access to highly active antiretroviral therapy (HAART), changing HIV infection from an invariably lethal disease into a chronic condition.

Regardless of the obvious benefits of antiretroviral drugs, 40% of patients experience failure on their first line of treatment, meaning that the virus replicates during therapy (Kaufmann et al., 2004). Each consecutive regimen again has a failure rate of 30–35% (Kaufmann et al., 2004). The reason for therapy failure is low plasma levels of antiretroviral drugs, caused by drug interactions, pharmacokinetic characteristics of the individual patient or insufficient patient adherence. Low drugs levels in plasma bring about drug resistance of the virus.

Patients who have experienced therapy failure are at risk of harboring and transmitting resistant virus.

This chapter will go into more detail about antiretroviral drugs, the development of HIV resistance against antiretroviral drugs, the transmission of resistant viruses and its implications for public health.

Antiretroviral Drugs

Antiretroviral drugs inhibit the viral proteins reverse transcriptase and protease. There are three main groups of antiretroviral drugs:
1. nucleoside-analogue reverse transcriptase inhibitors (NRTIs),

2. non-nucleoside reverse transcriptase inhibitors (NNRTIs), and
3. protease inhibitors (PIs).

Highly active antiretroviral therapy (HAART) aims to suppress viral replication. It consists of at least 3 drugs, generally from 2 different classes (triple therapy). Using triple therapy importantly reduces the rate of development of resistance.

Many treatment schemes consist of a number of pills that need to be taken according to a strict time schedule. The number of pills may vary from only 2 to over 15 per day. As far as we know now, the medication needs to be maintained life-long and can cause considerable side effects. These factors make adherence to therapy extremely difficult (Trotta et al., 2002).

Nevertheless, adherence is of the utmost importance for the success of the regimen. A study revealed that of the patients who took less than 80% of their prescribed drugs, 80% failed. In patients who took more than 95% of the pills the failure rate was 22% (Paterson et al., 2000).

Mechanisms of Resistance in HIV

Quick Replication and Replication Infidelity

Human immunodeficiency virus (HIV) is a retrovirus. Its genetic code is carried on double-stranded RNA. Reverse transcriptase (RT) is the enzyme that transcribes the RNA into DNA.

This RT lacks the ability to "proof-read": it is unable to correct the mistakes that have been made in the process of transcription. Thus RT is responsible for the low replication fidelity that is a feature of all human retroviruses. The mutation rate is in the order of 1 per 10^4 nucleotides, which means one mutation for each RNA copy (Colgrove and Japour, 1999). The HIV replicates at a very high rate; per day 1 to 10 billion new virus particles are produced.

Every virus particle contains two copies of RNA. This means that each day 2 to 20 billion mutations occur. Combined with the replication infidelity, this causes an enormous genetic diversity of the virus. A patient is not infected with just one virus, but with a heterogeneous "swarm" of viruses: a quasi-species of numerous slightly different viruses.

Fitness

The genetic variants of HIV have differences in their ability to replicate: their fitness. In the absence of drugs, the wild type virus is the fittest and therefore the dominant virus in the quasi-species. If viral replication in the presence of drugs continues, there is selection in favor of the viruses that are the least susceptible to the drug. They continue to replicate and manage to become the dominant species. Because of the rapid replication and the high mutation rate, this process of resistance can occur very quickly. In order to prevent the development of resistance, it is vital to suppress virus replication as much as possible.

In HAART at least 3 drugs are combined. This increases the genetic barrier to resistance: the viral population needs to collect a number of point mutations, before susceptibility to the drug regimen diminishes.

It is assumed that the viral population acquires resistance mutations at the cost of losing some of its replication fitness. When the selection pressure of the drug is removed, wild type virus will regain dominance and replace the resistant strain. However, the resistant viruses do not completely disappear. They stay present in the DNA of dormant memory T-cells of the patient as a genetic "archive" of mutant viruses (Finzi et al., 1997). Whenever the selective pressure of the drug is reintroduced, the resistant viruses will reappear in the plasma.

Failing HAART

Occurrence of resistance in a patient can be both the cause and the result of failing HAART.

Suboptimal plasma concentrations of drugs allow for ongoing virus replication, resulting in the selection of variants with reduced susceptibility to the drugs. These variants will form the dominant species.

Compartmentalization

It has been observed that the various compartments of the human body harbor HIV populations that are different from the ones in blood. Also the penetration of antiretroviral drugs may not be the same in the different compartments. Protease inhibitors, for instance, bind strongly to proteins. Decreased penetration of drugs has especially been observed in the central nervous system, genital tissues and in lymphoid tissue – so-called "sanctuary sites". The concentration of drugs is found to be lower and sometimes sub-therapeutic in these tissues. This may promote the emergence of resistant virus in sanctuary sites.

Transmitted Resistance: Consequences for Therapy and Disease Progression

People on HAART who have developed viral drug resistance can infect other people with resistant HIV strains. When a patient has been infected with a resistant virus, his virus is not fully susceptible to drugs when first starting antiretroviral therapy. In a study in the USA from 2002 the response to therapy was found to be worse in patients with primary resistance. After initiating HAART, the time to viral suppression was found to be significantly prolonged compared to patients with susceptible virus. In cases of viral relapse, the time to virologic failure was notably shorter in patients with resistant virus (Little et al., 2002).

It can be useful to perform baseline genotyping of the earliest possible plasma sample before initiating HAART, so that the most effective first regimen can be selected. Whether this is warranted or not depends on the incidence of primary resistance in the population.

Diagnosis of Resistance: Genotyping, Phenotyping

There are two types of assays that can be used to detect resistance of a virus: genotyping and phenotyping. Both techniques are costly and time-consuming. They can only be performed in specialized laboratories.

Genotypic Assays

A mutation is a change in the nucleotide sequence that can lead to a modification in the amino acid sequence of a protein. For example, a mutation in the 41st codon from ATG to TTG will result in a substitution of the amino acid methionine (M) with leucine (L). This is reported as "M41 L".

Mutations result in resistance of the virus to a specific drug. The base sequence of HIV, isolated from the patient, is compared to the sequence of a wild type reference laboratory strain. This enables identification of resistance-related mutations.

In a genotypic analysis the genome of HIV from the patient is isolated and the protease and reverse transcriptase genes are amplified by polymerase chain reaction (PCR). Then the nucleotide sequence of the protease and part of the reverse transcriptase are analyzed. In general, genotypic analysis is not possible when the viral load is less than 500 copies/mL. Mutations that are present in 10% or more of the virus population are detected. The assay is relatively difficult to perform and to interpret.

For the interpretation of the test result extensive knowledge is necessary about the relation between the genetic mutations and the drug susceptibility of the virus.

Phenotypic Assays

In this type of assay the *in vitro* susceptibility of the virus to an antiretroviral drug in cell culture is measured. The test is performed using recombinant viruses. The genome of the patient's virus is isolated and amplified by PCR. The RT and PR genes are then recombined with laboratory strains from which the RT and protease genes have been deleted. The susceptibility of these recombinant viruses to different drugs is measured as the IC_{50} and IC_{90} values, the concentrations at which respectively 50% and 90% of viral replication is inhibited compared to a susceptible reference strain. A disadvantage is that the assay is very time-consuming and costly. Only a few laboratories are able to perform the test (Hirsch and Richman, 2000).

Subtypes

There are various subtypes of HIV-1. They all originate from Central Africa, where the virus was introduced by monkeys into the human population in various places as subtypes (Rambaut et al., 2001). In Europe, North America and Australia the most prevalent subtype is B (70% in Europe). Worldwide the most prevalent subtypes are A and C.

The subtypes are based on differences in the base sequences of the RNA. The prevalence of resistance mutations is highest in subtype B. Being the most prevalent form in the Western world, this subtype has been exposed to antiretroviral therapy for a long time.

Some secondary resistance-related mutations may be present as natural polymorphisms in non-B subtypes.

There are non-B subtypes that have specific evolutionary pathways for developing drug resistance. Therefore the regular algorithms for detecting resistance in genotypic assays may not be reliable for non-B subtypes (Wensing et al., 2003).

Transmitted Drug Resistance

Before the introduction of HAART in 1995, patients used mono or dual therapy. These regimens were often not able to fully suppress viral replication, therefore resistance in treated patients occurred frequently. In 1993 a case of resistance to zidovudine was described in a patient who had not yet been exposed to the drug. This was the first described case of transmitted resistant HIV (Erice et al., 1993).

Nowadays there are numerous reports of transmitted resistance, in Europe more than 10% of therapy-naïve HIV-infected people showed resistance to at least one drug (Wensing and Boucher, 2003). A study from San Francisco over the period 1996–2001 even reported an alarming 23.5% in a high-risk population with a high proportion of white homosexual males – a group that has been heavily exposed to antiretroviral drugs (Grant et al., 2002). Other studies in the general population of the USA found percentages that were comparable to the percentages in Europe (Weinstock et al., 2004).

When a patient is newly infected, usually only a small number of virus particles has been transmitted. This small number will establish the new infection and grow out to form a new quasi-species. Therefore, newly infected people harbor a more homogeneous virus population than people who have been infected for a longer period.

In patients who have been infected with a resistant virus for some time, resistance sometimes cannot be detected anymore, because the resistant virus has mutated back to the wild type. This process is called "reversion to wild type". In case the virus needs a series of mutations in order to revert, mutations that are intermediates in this evolutionary pathway may give a clue for transmitted resistance. The originally transmitted resistant virus will nevertheless stay present in the dormant T cells of the patient.

Recent studies reveal that in some cases primary drug resistance can remain detectable for a longer period (Barbour et al., 2004). This can happen in a patient who has been infected with a (multi-drug) resistant virus only and consequently has no archived wild type virus. The virus has resistance-related mutations that impair the replication capacity to such extent that viral evolution occurs only very slowly or not at all (Brenner et al., 2002).

Transmission Fitness

Different groups of researchers compared the prevalence of resistance in patients experiencing virologic failure on HAART (the possible transmitters of resistance) with the prevalence of resistance in patients with primary HIV infection. They concluded that resistant HIV was transmitted 30% less frequently than the wild type virus from individuals who harbored drug resistance. The decreased rate of transmission that they found could not be explained by lower viral loads in the potential transmitters (Leigh Brown et al., 2003; Yerly et al., 2004).

So in addition to impaired replication fitness, it seems that the resistant virus also has a transmission disadvantage. However, the high reported prevalence of primary resistance leaves no doubt about whether a resistant virus can be infectious.

The Role of Primary HIV Infection (PHI) in Transmission of Resistance

Transmission of HIV is strongly related to the viral load in blood and in genital secretions. Patients with PHI are thought to be a very important factor in the spread of HIV (both drug-resistant and drug-sensitive), because at this stage of the disease many patients are unaware of their infection but the viral loads in their blood and genital fluids are already very high. This makes them highly infective. In a Swiss study phylogenetic analysis and contact tracing was performed in patients with PHI. The results showed that one-third of these patients were most likely infected by people who themselves had been infected only recently (Yerly et al., 2001).

Risk Groups for Transmitting Resistance

Transmission of resistant virus occurs in all transmission groups. Obviously both homosexual and heterosexual partners of HIV-infected people who receive HAART have an increased risk of becoming infected with resistant HIV.

Intravenous drug users on HAART are at high risk of developing drug resistance. Their lifestyle almost invariably conflicts with the strict rules for taking their antiretroviral drugs at set times and in combination with food (Zaccarelli et al., 2002). Their sexual partners, and the persons who share their needles, are therefore also at risk of contracting resistant HIV.

Finally, healthcare workers are another group at risk of being infected with resistant virus by their patients.

Vertical Transmission

Mother-to-child transmission (MTCT) of HIV can occur in the uterus, during delivery and during breast-feeding. In the absence of any treatment to prevent MTCT the risk of transmission in Europe is between 13 and 18% (Anon, 1991; Gabiano et al., 1992). In resource-limited areas this percentage is higher.

The use of antiretrovirals to prevent MTCT started in the early 1990s. In 1994 the remarkable results of a clinical study were published in which zidovudine was administered to the mother during pregnancy and labor and to the newborn in the first 6 weeks of life. In the group that received zidovudine only 7.6% of the babies were infected with HIV as compared to 22.6% in the placebo group (Connor et al., 1994).

Since then many different schemes have been used that reduced the rate of MTCT: a short course of zidovudine, combinations of zidovudine and lamivudine, single oral doses of nevirapine given to the mother at the onset of labor and to the newborn in the first 48–72 hours. All these regimens, however, confer resistance. The first reported case of a neonate with zidovudine-resistant HIV was in 1994 (Siegrist et al., 1994). Especially drugs like nevirapine and lamivudine can induce resistance very rapidly, because only one single mutation is enough to make the virus highly resistant to the drug.

Nowadays, the risk of transmitting the virus to the fetus is less than 2%. Therefore, treatment with HAART should be considered in every pregnant woman, regardless of her CD4 count (Watts, 2002).

In resource-limited settings treatment for the prevention of MTCT is often based on zidovudine alone or a combination of zidovudine during pregnancy combined with a single dose of nevirapine during delivery. However, a recent study from Thailand showed that in women who started nevirapine-based triple therapy after delivery, a history of a single intrapartum dose of nevirapine was associated with a significant decrease in the rate of virological suppression at 6 months (Jourdain et al., 2004).

Also during HAART resistance can develop and MTCT of resistant virus has been described. In 2001 the first case of vertically transmitted multidrug-resistant virus was reported (Johnson et al., 2001). It can be assumed that the therapeutic options for a newborn that has been vertically infected with a resistant virus are limited. Resistance testing in the pregnant woman and adjustment of antenatal therapy on the basis of the resistance profile can limit the risk of vertical transmission of resistant virus.

Post-Exposure Prophylaxis and Resistance

In case of accidental exposure to HIV, the matter of resistance needs to be taken into consideration when prescribing post-exposure prophylaxis (PEP). In 1998 and 1999, 41 source patients of needle-stick injuries in the United States were genotyped. More than 40% of them carried a primary mutation that was associated with resistance (Gerberding, 2003). Despite the use of PEP after occupational exposure, transmission of resistant strains of HIV has been described (Anon, 2001).

Resistance testing of the source patient takes too long to be helpful in deciding which PEP regimen should be started, as PEP should be started within a few hours after exposure. It is useful to take the treatment history of the source patient into account in order to predict the mutations that might be present. If available, earlier viral genotypes of the source patient can provide the necessary information. If this information is not available, it is advised to start a standard PEP regimen and to adjust it – if necessary – when additional information becomes available.

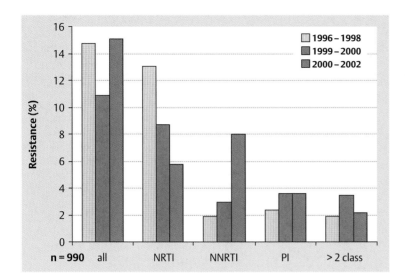

Fig. 3.**1** Time trends in recently infected patients in Europe, the CATCH study (by courtesy of A. M. Wensing).

Epidemiology

Measuring Transmission of Resistance

Surveillance is necessary to monitor the pattern of an epidemic. Is the incidence rising or falling? Is there a shift in populations at risk?

To get reliable answers one needs to select the appropriate study population. In studying the prevalence of transmitted resistance of HIV, this is a subject of much debate.

In antiretroviral-naïve patients who have been infected long ago, it can be difficult to find evidence of primary resistance. The resistant virus may have reverted to the wild type. The resistant virus will, however, be present in the dormant memory CD4 T cells, and therefore may escape detection by genotyping.

Ideally, incidence studies are performed in a population of seroconverters. However, these patients are difficult to identify and the group that is identified may not represent the total seroconverter population. The identified group may be biased as it consists on the one hand of people who had clinical symptoms of primary HIV infection and on the other hand of frequent testers – possibly people with higher than average risk behavior (Tang and Pillay, 2004).

An alternative is to study the incidence of primary resistance in newly diagnosed patients. The advantage is that the identified group will be bigger. A disadvantage is that much time may have elapsed since infection and mutations may have disappeared in the meantime. However, recent studies indicate that reversion is a slow process (Little et al., 2003).

The most practical group to study is the group of newly diagnosed patients. Nevertheless, as a result of reversion to wild type the measured prevalence in this group may be too low.

Public Health Impact

There is a huge variety between populations in the prevalence of transmitted resistance, but in general its prevalence seems to be increasing (Little et al., 2002; Grant et al., 2002).

An important factor is the population's level of exposure to antiretroviral drugs. In a population with a high proportion of homosexual males in San Francisco, where antiretrovirals have been widely available for many years, the prevalence of primary resistance in recently infected people was found to be as high as 23.5% (Grant et al., 2002). Conversely, samples from recently infected patients from Seattle and Los Angeles showed a prevalence of 7% (Sullivan et al., 2002).

A problem in evaluating the spread of resistant virus is the methodological heterogeneity of the various studies that renders them not well comparable. The inclusion criteria may not be the same, different interpretations of the genotypes may have been used, or there may have been differences in which mutations were considered major and minor. In order to get a clear picture of the ep-

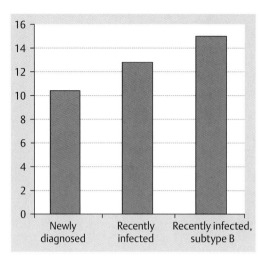

Fig. 3.**2**   Baseline resistance in the CATCH study: newly diagnosed subjects: 10.4%; recently infected: 12.8%; recently infected subtype B: 15% (by courtesy of A. M. Wensing).

idemiology of primary resistance, it is vital to analyze the available data in a standardized manner.

An important initiative was the CATCH study; combined analysis of resistance transmission over time of chronically and acute infected HIV patients in Europe. This study looked retrospectively at the prevalence of genotypic drug resistance among antiretroviral naïve patients in Europe in the period between 1996 and 2002. A total of 2208 patients from 29 countries was included in the study. This study showed that 10.4% of all drug-naïve patients carried one or more resistance-related mutations. In recently infected patients who were infected with subtype B the percentage of primary resistance was as high as 15% (Fig. 3.**2**).

Especially the group of recently infected patients revealed an important increase in the prevalence of primary resistance (Fig. 3.**1**). In the period from 1996 to 1999, 17% of recently infected people harbored one or more resistance-related mutations. In the period from 2000 to 2002 this was a distressing 28% (Wensing et al., 2003).

CATCH was a substudy of the SPREAD program (Strategy to Control SPREAD of HIV Drug Resistance) supported by the European Commission (project number: OJ1999/C361/06). In this project clinicians, virologists and epidemiologists from 18 European countries are working together to collect patient information in a systematic manner and to perform genotypic analysis of the virus in a network of quality controlled reference laboratories throughout Europe. The data will be stored in a large database and analyzed using mathematical models. The results will be used to identify risk groups and to predict future trends. One of the final aims is to develop a strategy to control the transmission of drug-resistant HIV.

Surveillance of transmitted resistance is also necessary on a worldwide scale. New initiatives in this field have been launched recently:

❖ WATCH (Worldwide Analysis of resistance Transmission over time of Chronically and acute infected HIV patients) is the worldwide continuation of CATCH; it collects and analyzes retrospectively genotypic sequences of antiretroviral naïve patients from all over the world.

❖ UNITEMORE (UNiformity In TEsting and MOnitoring HIV REsistance) is initiated by WHO and SPREAD and supported by the European Commission (project number: P516030).

The latter has aims similar to those of SPREAD, but focuses on surveillance of HIV resistance throughout the world. The activities of UNITEMORE can be divided into three main areas:
1. coordinating the selection, establishment and validation of national HIV-drug resistance surveillance teams in over 40 countries in Eastern Europe, Africa, Asia and Latin and South America,
2. developing common clinical laboratory standards for the monitoring of HIV resistance (standard protocols, sample collection methods and standard data storage and analysis), and
3. coordinating training and operational support of the countries' HIV drug resistance surveillance teams.

Discussion

Transmission of resistant HIV is a growing public health problem. It significantly limits therapeutic options and unfavorably influences the treatment outcome.

Prevention of transmission of resistance is vital. First of all, to prevent the development of resistance in the patient who receives HAART, monitoring of therapy response, adjusting therapy on the basis of a genotypic resistance profile in the case of virologic failure and encouraging the patient to adhere to the therapy are very important.

Patients who receive HAART have extensive contact with healthcare providers and thus are easily available for education on the prevention of transmission. It is the task of healthcare providers working in HIV to put extensive efforts into educating their patients on safe sex, risk behavior and their responsibility to prevent the transmission of (resistant) virus. Even if plasma levels are low or undetectable, the viral load in genital secretions may be higher, due to compartmentalization.

Because people may have been infected with resistant HIV in the first place, baseline genotyping – before starting therapy – may be indicated, depending on the incidence of transmitted resistance in the population. The antiretroviral regimen should be based on the resistance profile of the virus.

Surveillance of transmission of (multi)drug-resistant virus in a standardized manner enables us to make timely adjustments to treatment policies and to intervene where necessary. SPREAD is an important European project to identify risk groups and predict future trends. The final aim is to develop a strategy to control the transmission of drug-resistant HIV.

References

Anon. Children born to women with HIV-1 infection: natural history and risk of transmission. European Collaborative Study. Lancet 1991; 337: 253–260

Anon. U. S. Public Health Service Guidelines for the management of occupational exposures to HBV, HCV, and HIV and recommendations for postexposure prophylaxis. MMWR Recomm Rep 2001; 50: 1–52

Barbour JD, Hecht FM, Wrin T, Liegler TJ, Ramstead CA, Busch MP, Segal MR, Petropoulos CJ, Grant RM. Persistence of primary drug resistance among recently HIV-1 infected adults. AIDS 2004; 18: 1683–1689

Brenner BG, Routy JP, Petrella M, Moisi D, Oliveira M, Detorio M, Spira B, Essabag V, Conway B, Lalonde R, Sekaly RP, Wainberg MA. Persistence and fitness of multidrug-resistant human immunodeficiency virus type 1 acquired in primary infection. J Virol 2002; 76: 1753–1761

Colgrove R, Japour A. A combinatorial ledge: reverse transcriptase fidelity, total body viral burden, and the implications of multiple-drug HIV therapy for the evolution of antiviral resistance. Antiviral Res 1999; 41: 45–56

Connor EM, Sperling RS, Gelber R, Kiselev P, Scott G, O'Sullivan MJ, VanDyke R, Bey M, Shearer W, Jacobson RL. Reduction of maternal-infant transmission of human immunodeficiency virus type 1 with zidovudine treatment. Pediatric AIDS Clinical Trials Group Protocol 076 Study Group. N Engl J Med 1994; 331: 1173–1180

Erice A, Mayers DL, Strike DG, Sannerud KJ, McCutchan FE, Henry K, Balfour Jr HH. Brief report: primary infection with zidovudine-resistant human immunodeficiency virus type 1. N Engl J Med 1993; 328: 1163–1165

Finzi D, Hermankova M, Pierson T, Carruth LM, Buck C, Chaisson RE, Quinn TC, Chadwick K, Margolick J, Brookmeyer R, Gallant J, Markowitz M, Ho DD, Richman DD, Siliciano RF. Identification of a reservoir for HIV-1 in patients on highly active antiretroviral therapy. Science 1997; 278: 1295–1300

Gabiano C, Tovo P A, de Martino M, Galli L, Giaquinto C, Loy A, Schoeller MC, Giovannini M, Ferranti G, Rancilio L. Mother-to-child transmission of human immunodeficiency virus type 1: risk of infection and correlates of transmission. Pediatrics 1992; 90: 369–374

Gerberding JL. Clinical practice. Occupational exposure to HIV in health care settings. N Engl J Med 2003; 348: 826–833

Grant RM, Hecht FM, Warmerdam M, Liu L, Liegler T, Petropoulos CJ, Hellmann NS, Chesney M, Busch MP, Kahn JO. Time trends in primary HIV-1 drug resistance among recently infected persons. JAMA 2002; 288: 181–188

Hirsch MS, Richman DD. The role of genotypic resistance testing in selecting therapy for HIV. JAMA 2000; 284: 1649–1650

Johnson VA, Petropoulos CJ, Woods CR, Hazelwood JD, Parkin NT, Hamilton CD, Fiscus SA. Vertical transmission of multidrug-resistant human immunodeficiency virus type 1 (HIV-1) and continued evolution of drug resistance in an HIV-1-infected infant. J Infect Dis 2001; 183: 1688–1693

Jourdain G, Ngo-Giang-Huong N, Le Coeur S, Bowonwatanuwong C, Kantipong P, Leechanachai P, Ariyadej S, Leenasirimakul P, Hammer S, Lallemant M. Intrapartum exposure to nevirapine and subsequent maternal responses to nevirapine-based antiretroviral therapy. N Engl J Med 2004; 351: 229–240

Kaufmann GR, Khanna N, Weber R, Perrin L, Furrer H, Cavassini M, Ledergerber B, Vernazza P, Bernasconi E, Rickenbach M, Hirschel B, Battegay M. Long-term virological response to multiple sequential regimens of highly active antiretroviral therapy for HIV infection. Antivir Ther 2004; 9: 263–274

Leigh Brown AJ, Frost SD, Mathews WC, Dawson K, Hellmann NS, Daar ES, Richman DD, Little SJ. Transmission fitness of drug-resistant human immunodeficiency virus and the prevalence of resistance in the antiretroviral-treated population. J Infect Dis 2003; 187: 683–686

Little SJ, Holte S, Routy JP, Daar ES, Markowitz M, Collier AC, Koup RA, Mellors JW, Connick E, Conway B, Kilby M, Wang L, Whitcomb JM, Hellmann NS, Richman DD. Antiretroviral-drug resistance among patients recently infected with HIV. N Engl J Med 2002; 347: 385–394

Little SJ, Dawson K, Hellmann NS, Richman DD, Frost SDW. Persistence of transmitted drug-resistant virus among subjects with primary HIV infection deferring antiretroviral therapy. Antivir Ther 2003; 8: S115

Paterson DL, Swindells S, Mohr J, Brester M, Vergis EN, Squier C, Wagener MM, Singh N. Adherence to protease inhibitor therapy and outcomes in patients with HIV infection. Ann Intern Med 2000; 133: 21–30

Rambaut A, Robertson DL, Pybus OG, Peeters M, Holmes EC. Human immunodeficiency virus. Phylogeny and the origin of HIV-1. Nature 2001; 410: 1047–1048

Siegrist CA, Yerly S, Kaiser L, Wyler CA, Perrin L. Mother to child transmission of zidovudine-resistant HIV-1. Lancet 1994; 344: 1771–1772

Sullivan PS, Buskin SE, Turner JH, Cheingsong R, Saekhou A, Kalish ML, Jones JL, Respess R, Kovacs A, Heneine W. Low prevalence of antiretroviral resistance among persons recently infected with human immunodeficiency virus in two US cities. Int J STD AIDS 2002; 13: 554–558

Tang JW, Pillay D. Transmission of HIV-1 drug resistance. J Clin Virol 2004; 30: 1–10

Trotta MP, Ammassari A, Melzi S, Zaccarelli M, Ladisa N, Sighinolfi L, Mura MS, d'Arminio Monforte A, Antinori A. Treatment-related factors and highly active antiretroviral therapy adherence. J Acquir Immune Defic Syndr 2002; 31 (Suppl 3): S128–S131

Watts DH. Management of human immunodeficiency virus infection in pregnancy. N Engl J Med 2002; 346: 1879–1891

Weinstock HS, Zaidi I, Heneine W, Bennett D, Garcia-Lerma JG, Douglas Jr JM, LaLota M, Dickinson G, Schwarcz S, Torian L, Wendell D, Paul S, Goza GA, Ruiz J, Boyett B, Kaplan JE. The epidemiology of antiretroviral drug resistance among drug-naive HIV-1-infected persons in 10 US cities. J Infect Dis 2004; 189: 2174–2180

Wensing AM, Boucher CA. Worldwide transmission of drug-resistant HIV. AIDS Rev 2003; 5: 140–155

Wensing AMJ, van de Vijver DAMC, Asjo B, Balotta C, Camacho R, de Mendoza C, Deroo S, Derdelinckx I, Grossman Z, Hamouda O, Hatzakis A, Hoepelman IM, Horban A, Korn K, Kucherer C, Nielsen C, Ormaasen V, Perrin L, Paraskevis D, Puchhammer E, Roman F, Salminen M, Schmit JCC, Soriano V, Stanczak G, Stanojevic M, Vandamme A-M, Van Laethem K, Violin M, Yerly S, Zazzi M, Boucher CAB and on behalf of the SPREAD programme. Prevalence of transmitted drug resistance in Europe is largely influenced by the presence of non-b sequences: analysis of 1400 patients from 16 countries: the CATCH-study. Antivir Ther 2003; 8: S131

Yerly S, Vora S, Rizzardi P, Chave JP, Vernazza PL, Flepp M, Telenti A, Battegay M, Veuthey AL, Bru JP, Rickenbach M, Hirschel B, Perrin L. Acute HIV infection: impact on the spread of HIV and transmission of drug resistance. AIDS 2001; 15: 2287–2292

Yerly S, Jost S, Telenti A, Flepp M, Kaiser L, Chave JP, Vernazza P, Battegay M, Furrer H, Chanzy B, Burgisser P, Rickenbach M, Gebhardt M, Bernard MC, Perneger T, Hirschel B, Perrin L. Infrequent transmission of HIV-1 drug-resistant variants. Antivir Ther 2004; 9: 375–384

Zaccarelli M, Barracchini A, De Longis P, Perno CF, Soldani F, Liuzzi G, Serraino D, Ippolito G, Antinori A. Factors related to virologic failure among HIV-positive injecting drug users treated with combination antiretroviral therapy including two nucleoside reverse transcriptase inhibitors and nevirapine. AIDS Patient Care STDS 2002; 16: 67–73

3.2 Management of Primary HIV Infection in Germany. Preliminary Data from Two German Cohorts

C. Kögl, E. Wolf, A. Goetzenich, H. Jessen, K. Schewe,
M. Freiwald, J. Goelz, H. Knechten, H. Jaeger

Participating Centers

Prof. Dr. M. Althoff, Bürgerhospital Frankfurt, Germany; Dr. W. Becker, München, Germany; Dr. I. Becker-Boost, Duisburg, Germany; Dr. D. Berzow, Hamburg, Germany; Dr. B. Bieniek, Berlin, Germany; Drs. J. Brust, D. Schuster, Mannheim, Germany; Dr. S. Dupke, Berlin, Germany; Dr. A. Dix, Klinikum Konstanz, Germany; Dr. S. Fenske, Hamburg, Germany; Drs. M. Freiwald, M. Rausch, Berlin, Germany; Dr. H. Gellermann, Hamburg, Germany; Dr. A. Hammond, Klinikum Augsburg, Germany; Dr. B. Hintsche, Berlin, Germany; Dr. C. Hoffmann, HIV-Ambulanz der Uniklinik Kiel, Germany; Drs. H. Jäger, E. Jägel-Guedes, München, Germany; Dr. H. Jessen, Berlin, Germany; Dr. J. Gölz, Berlin, Germany; Dr. J. Koelzsch, Berlin, Germany; Prof. Dr. E. Helm, Dr. G. Knecht, IFs Frankfurt, Germany; Dr. H. Knechten, Aachen, Germany; Dr. M. Lademann, Universität Rostock; Drs. T. Locher, P. Gute, Frankfurt, Germany; Dr. S. Mauruschat, Wuppertal, Germany; Dr. S. Mauss, Düsseldorf, Germany; Dr. V. Miasnikov, Düsseldorf, Germany; Dr. F. Mosthaf, Karlsruhe, Germany; Dr. B. Reuter, Berlin, Germany; Dr. B. Ross, Universitätsklinium der GHS Essen, Germany; Dr. H. Schalk, Wien, Austria; Dr. B. Schappert, Mainz, Germany; Dr. E. Schnaitmann, Stuttgart, Germany; Dr. L. Schneider, Fürth, Germany; Dr. A. Schneidewind, Uniklinik Regensburg, Germany; Dr. W. Schüler-Maué, Berlin, Germany; Dr. C. Schuler, Berlin, Germany; Dr. W. Starke, Wiesbaden, Germany; Drs. A. Ulmer, M. Müller, Stuttgart, Germany; Drs A. Weitner, K. Schewe, Hamburg, Germany; Dr. C. Zamani, Hannover, Germany

Introduction

The diagnosis of primary/acute human immunodeficiency virus (HIV) infection (PHI) tends to occur relatively late; quite often several consultations are needed to arrive at this diagnosis (Weintrob et al., 2002).

The viral set point is usually reached approximately six months after infection with HIV; initial HIV plasma concentrations are often very high (up to 100 million copies/mL). The viral set point level seems to predict the risk of progression of HIV infection to clinical disease and ultimately death (Musey et al., 1997). Through treatment of acute HIV infection with highly active antiretroviral therapy (HAART), a broader HIV-specific immune response can be maintained and the virus replication can be controlled (Oxenius et al., 2000; Rosenberg et al., 2000). A comparable effect of early therapy in combination with structured therapy interruptions was shown in animal testing (Lori et al., 2000), as well as in a small patient cohort (Altfeld et al., 2000; Hermans et al., 2001). An example of ideal virus control is seen in the "Berlin patient". Antiretroviral therapy was started in the acute phase of an HIV infection with two treatment interruptions. During the second 16-day interruption no rebound in viral load could be detected. Stopping HAART after approximately six months did not lead to an increase in viral load nor to negative immunological effects in a follow-up of several years (Lisziewicz et al., 1999).

The goal of an immediate start of therapy during or even before seroconversion is to increase immunological control and hence to reduce disease progression. After a few months of effective therapy, treatment could possibly be interrupted and eventually stopped completely.

The objective of two nation-wide German cohorts is to evaluate treatment strategies and outcomes in acute HIV infection.

Primary HIV Infections (PHI) – Background

Bruce Walker and his group, who initially investigated very early treatment of PHI, stressing structured treatment interruptions to boost cytotoxic T-cell and HIV-specific CD4 cell responses, questioned an early therapy start and the resulting benefit of immunological virus control (Walker et al., 2003; Connors, 2003; Kaufmann et al., 2004). Preliminary study results were, in part, presented at CROI 2003 and CROI 2004 (Hoen et al., 2004). Even with early treatment, only very few patients seem to gain control over their virus (Kinloch et al., 2003; Lafeuillade et al., 2003; Goujard et al., 2003). The majority of patients cannot maintain suppression of viremia after a sequence of HAART and structured treatment interruptions (Lacabaratz-Porret et al., 2004). Successful virus suppression was not dependent on the use of three versus more antiretroviral agents or on the use of protease inhibitors (Grey et al., 2003; Lafeuillade et al., 2003). The only controlled (non-randomized) study was unable to demonstrate a conclusive benefit of treatment (Hecht et al., 2003). In the SEROCO cohort, early treatment did not lead to lower viral load levels after interruption of effective HAART regimen (Desquilbet et al., 2004). Lower baseline viral load (< 50,000) and a shorter time to viral suppression on therapy (< 16 weeks) were predictive for a longer time to viral load rebound (Smith et al., 2004).

Prime-DAG

Prime-DAG is a DAGNAE (German Association of Physicians in Private Practice) project to investigate treatment strategies in acute HIV infection. The project was created in response to questions posed by DAGNAE members, and is aimed at improving PHI awareness and at devising a tool for guiding diagnosis and therapy. Prime-DAG is a nation-wide, multi-centric, 24-month cohort evaluation. It is purely observational with no randomization. Every individual treatment with or without treatment interruptions as well as non-treatment are recorded. Prime-DAG was started in July 2001 with a focus on early treatment of PHI, as suggested by scientific data at that time.

Prime-DAG: Inclusion Criteria

In this evaluation patients from 24 centers with symptomatic or asymptomatic HIV primary infection diagnosed after 1 July 2001 were included. Criteria for primary HIV infection were either
❖ a negative ELISA coupled with a detectable plasma viral load, or
❖ a documented Western blot with less than 5 bands, or
❖ a negative HIV test within three months before seroconversion.

Treatment should have been started either before seroconversion or no later than 12 weeks after seroconversion.

Any form of treatment or non-treatment was acceptable. One recommendation was the use of zidovudine, lamivudine and lopinavir/ritonavir for 8 months followed by a stop in therapy (Clotet, 2004). Another conceivable possibility was to treat for at least three months until viral load was below the limit of detection, then continue with alternating cycles of 2-week interruptions and 4-week treatment phases.

Prime-DAG: Cohort and Results

One hundred patients were included from 22 private clinics and 2 hospital ambulatory care centers. Ninety-five were men and 5 were women, ranging in age from 18 to 62 years (mean: 35 years). Eighty-one patients stated homosexual contacts as their transmission risk, 11 patients stated heterosexual contacts, 1 patient injection drug use; for 7 patients the risk was unknown.

In 90 patients (90%), clinical symptoms with or without known risk for transmission were the reason for HIV testing. Four asymptomatic patients

Table 3.1   Main symptoms

Symptom	N	%
Fever	75	75
Lymphadenopathy	59	59
Exanthema	38	38
Diarrhea	15	15
Pharyngitis, stomatitis, tonsillitis	10	10
Candida esophagitis	4	4

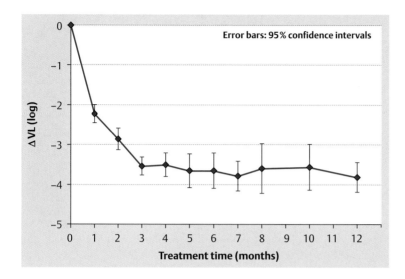

Fig. 3.**3** Mean changes in viral load during treatment with HAART in the Prime-DAG cohort.

Table 3.**2**   CD4 cell counts and initial viral load during seroconversion

	Mean	Median	Range
Absolute CD4 cell counts (1/µL)	542	460	132 – 1205
Relative CD4 cell counts (%)	24	23	4 – 46
Viral load (copies/mL)	4.4 mio	> 500 000	100 – 327 mio

(4%) stated unsafe sexual behavior within the last 3 months, one patient (1%) reported a needle stick injury, and 5 patients (5%) underwent routine testing.

The most common symptoms among the 100 acutely infected patients are shown in Table 3.**1**.

The first recorded viral load and the baseline CD4 cell counts are shown in Table 3.**2**. Ninety-two patients were treated with HAART during seroconversion or in the first 3 months after seroconversion. 8 patients remained untreated.

Eighty-one of the 92 treated patients received a triple combination, the remainder (n = 11) were prescribed 4 or more antiretroviral drugs. Seventy-six patients were treated with a combination of NRTI and PI, another 8 patients with a combination of NRTI and NNRTI and 8 patients exclusively with NRTI. Five patients started treatment before seroconversion (in these patients a detectable viral load was coupled with a negative ELISA), 53 patients started during and 34 patients within 12 weeks after seroconversion.

The median treatment time has been 7.9 months (range: 2.1 – 16.0 months). Twenty-three patients interrupted therapy: 12 once, 3 twice, and 8 patients three times or more. So far, 46 of the 92 patients have discontinued therapy. Figs. 3.**3** and 3.**4** show the decrease of viral load and the increase in absolute CD4 cell count during treatment of primary infection.

Early treatment of HIV infection was very effective. After 3 months the viral load was under the limit of detection (50 copies/mL) in 65% and after 6 months in 96% of the patients.

Ac-DAG

During the course of Prime-DAG, DAGNAE was able to create a database evaluating the treatment of primary HIV infection. Upon reaching this goal, there still seemed to be a continuing demand for more documentation in response to unanswered and new questions. Hence, DAGNAE started a follow-up project with another 100 patients to be documented over two years.

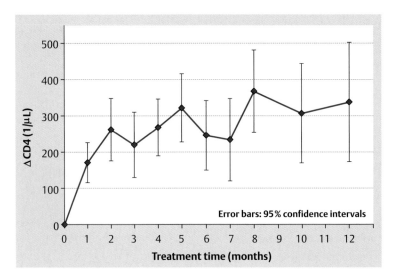

Fig. 3.**4**   Mean changes in absolute CD4 cell count during treatment with HAART in the Prime-DAG cohort.

Ac-DAG: Inclusion Criteria

Patients with symptomatic or asymptomatic HIV primary infection after 1 January 2003 were included. Criteria for primary HIV infection corresponded to the criteria used in Prime-DAG.

There were no treatment recommendations; every form of treatment including non-treatment was documented. The treatment decisions were in the hands of the treating physician and the patient.

Ac-DAG: Cohort

Ninety patients so far have been included from 36 private clinics and 4 hospital ambulatory care centers. Eighty-seven were men and 3 were women, ranging in age from 20 to 60 years (mean: 35 years). Seventy-five patients (83%) stated homosexual contacts as their transmission risk, 6 patients (7%) heterosexual contacts, 2 patients (2%) injection drug use; for 7 patients (8%) the risk was unknown.

In 76 patients (84%), clinical symptoms with or without known risk for transmission were the reason for HIV testing, 11 patients (12%) stated unsafe sexual behavior in the last 3 months as the reason for a test, and another 3 patients (3%) underwent routine testing.

Results

For all following analyses the Prime-DAG and Ac-DAG cohorts were pooled into one database.

One-hundred and ninety cases with primary HIV infection could be evaluated (182 males and 8 females). The median observation time up to the point of writing has been 17.9 months (range: 1.3 – 37.7 months). Eighty-seven percent of the patients presented with an acute retroviral syndrome (ARS). The main symptom was fever (76%), followed by lymphadenopathy (50%) and exanthema (40%). The initial recorded viral load and CD4 cell counts are shown in Table 3.**3**.

In patients with ARS, the median initial viral load was significantly higher than in patients without ARS ($\geq$ 500,000 versus 20,600 copies/mL). The median CD4 cell counts were 467/μL and 667/μL, respectively (see Table 3.**4**).

In 142 patients, treatment was started immediately, 48 patients remained untreated. One hundred and twenty-six of the 142 treated patients (89%) received a triple combination therapy and 16 patients (11%) a combination of four or more antiretroviral drugs. One hundred and twelve patients were treated with a combination of NRTI and PI, another 20 patients with a combination of NRTI and NNRTI and 10 patients exclusively with NRTI. An association was found between drug class use and CD4 cell counts and/or initial viral load (Table 3.**5**). Triple NRTI regimens were only used in the case of a relatively low viral load and a good CD4 cell count.

Table 3.**3**   Prime-DAG and Ac-DAG cohorts: CD4 cell counts and initial viral load during seroconversion

	Mean	Median	Range
Absolute CD4 cell counts (1/µL)	552	486	120–1543
Relative CD4 cell counts (%)	25	25	4–50
Viral load (copies/mL)	2.6 mio	399456	100–327 mio

Table 3.**4**   CD4 cells and initial viral load during seroconversion with respect to ARS

	With ARS (n = 23)		Without ARS (n = 167)		p value
	Median	Range	Median	Range	
Absolute CD4 cell counts (1/µL)	467	120–1342	667	246–1543	0.06
Relative CD4 cell counts (%)	25	4–50	34	16–42	0.004
Viral load (copies/mL)	500001	100–327 mio	20600	120–750000	<0.0001

Table 3.**5**   Treatment regimens, median CD4 cells and median viral load at baseline

	N	Viral load (copies/mL)	Abs. CD4 (1/µL)	Rel. CD4 (%)
Only NRTI	10	50400	674	25
NRTI + NNRTI	20	316432	507	16
NRTI + PI	112	477906	442	25

Eleven patients started treatment before seroconversion (in these patients a detectable viral load was coupled with a negative ELISA), 79 patients started during and 52 patients within 12 weeks after seroconversion. Twenty-five of 142 patients (18%) interrupted treatment: 14 once, 3 twice, and 8 patients three times or more.

Changes in viral load with respect to the number of drugs are shown in Fig. 3.**5**, those with respect to the treatment regimes in Fig. 3.**6** and those with respect to treatment start before, during or within 12 weeks after seroconversion can be seen in Fig. 3.**7**.

There were no significant differences in the decrease of the viral load or in the increase of CD4 cells

❖ between patients treated with three or four (or more) antiretroviral drugs,
❖ between patients treated with either only NRTI, with NRTI plus NNRTI, or with NRTI plus PI, and
❖ between patients treated before, during or within 12 weeks after seroconversion.

Sixty-two patients (25 with treatment interruptions) discontinued antiretroviral therapy after a median treatment time of 8.1 months (range 1.0–21.7 months).

At discontinuation, 43 patients (73%) had an undetectable viral load and 13 patients (21%) had a viral load below 400 copies/mL. The median absolute CD4 cell count was 789/µL and the median relative CD4 cell count was 37% (Table 3.**6**).

Fig. 3.**8** shows the viral load and Fig. 3.**9** the absolute CD4 cell counts after treatment stop.

Six months after discontinuation (n = 24) the median viral load showed an increase to 37,700 copies/mL (mean: 93,704 copies/mL; range: <50–750,000 copies/mL) and the median absolute CD4 cell counts a decrease to 627/µL. One year after treatment stop the viral load of two patients remained below detection. With respect to viral load and CD4 cell count after discontinuation, no differences could be detected between patients with or without treatment interruption, and be-

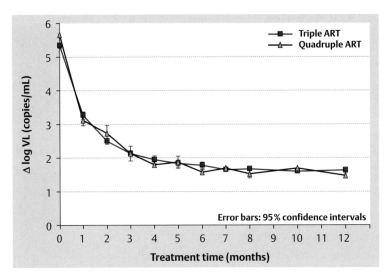

Fig. 3.**5** Mean changes in viral load during treatment with HAART with respect to the number of drugs.

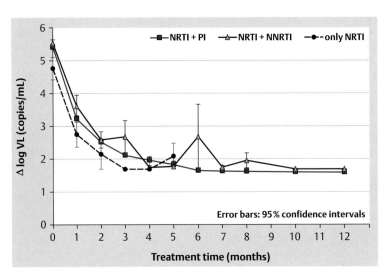

Fig. 3.**6** Mean changes in viral load during treatment with HAART with respect to the treatment regimens.

Table 3.**6** CD4 cells and viral load at treatment stop

	Mean	Median	Range
Absolute CD4 cell counts (1/µL)	804	789	394–1197
Relative CD4 cell counts (%)	36	37	16–55
Viral load (copies/mL)	290	<50	<50–7220

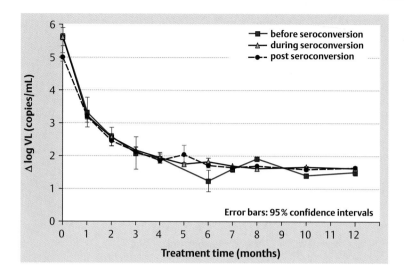

Fig. 3.**7** Mean changes in viral load during treatment with HAART with respect to treatment start before, during or within 12 weeks after seroconversion.

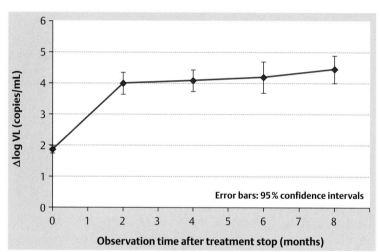

Fig. 3.**8** Mean changes in viral load after discontinuation of HAART in the Prime-DAG and Ac-DAG cohorts.

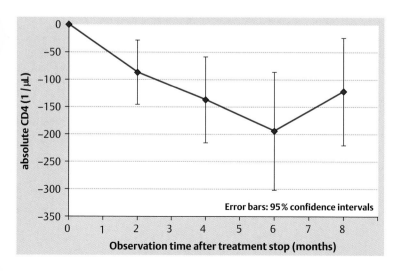

Fig. 3.**9** Mean changes in CD4 cell count after discontinuation of HAART in the Prime-DAG and Ac-DAG cohorts.

Table 3.**7**   CD4 cells and viral load in untreated patients

Viral load (copies/mL)	N	Mean	Median	Range
Base	48	440 130	215 000	463 – 6 mio
3 months after seroconversion	20	141 988	76 950	399 – 735 000
6 months after seroconversion	13	160 623	131 000	7395 – 750 000
Absolute CD4 cells [1/μL]		**Mean**	**Median**	**Range**
Base	48	640	572	246 – 1543
3 months after seroconversion	20	653	580	295 – 1543
6 months after seroconversion	13	550	569	241 – 1186

tween patients treated before, during or within 12 weeks after seroconversion.

The progression of viral load and absolute CD4 cell counts in untreated patients is shown in Table 3.**7**.

Prospects

From today's viewpoint, it is impossible to give a definite recommendation for treatment in primary HIV infections. The concept of early treatment with potential treatment interruptions may have its merits. It is possible that early treatment may result in a lower viral load set point.

In the cohorts Prime-DAG and Ac-DAG symptomatic primary HIV infection was associated with significantly higher viral load levels and lower CD4 cells. Patients with and without ARS responded favorably to early treatment.

Upon diagnosis of an acute HIV infection, physician and patient have to decide in the light of accessible data, whether or not antiretroviral treatment should be started as early as possible or delayed until a viral load set point is reached, immune deficiency has advanced or symptoms have developed. Scientific data on optimal management of primary HIV infection at this point in time are not conclusive.

Untreated patients have to be compared with patients on treatment in more detail before a decision can be reached whether to recommend early HAART in primary HIV infection or not.

Acknowledgements

Prime-DAG was made possible through the unconditional financial support from Abbott and GlaxoSmithKline.

Ac-DAG was made possible through the unconditional financial support from Abbott, Boehringer Ingelheim, Bristol-Myers Squibb, Gilead Sciences, GlaxoSmithKline, Hoffmann-La Roche and MSD Sharp & Dohme.

References

Altfeld M, Rosenberg ES, Eldridge RL et al. Increase in breadth and frequency of CTL responses after structured therapy interruptions in individuals treated with HAART during acute HIV-1 Infection. San Francisco: 7th Conference on Retroviruses and Opportunistic Infections, 2000: Abstract 357

Clotet B. Comparison of regimens as initial therapy for HIV. N Engl J Med 2004; 350: 1053 – 1054

Connors M. Shifting the paradigm of immunologic control of HIV. Boston: 10th Conference on Retroviruses and Opportunistic Infections, 2003: Abstract 165

Desquilbet L, Goujard C, Deveau C et al. HIV-1 RNA viral load dynamics after discontinuation of early and effective HAART initiated during primary HIV-1 infection. San Francisco: 11th Conference on Retroviruses and Opportunistic Infections, 2004: Abstract 397

Goujard C, Deveau C, Sinet M et al. Impact of therapeutic interruptions in patients treated during primary infection. Boston: 10th Conference on Retroviruses and Opportunistic Infections, 2003: Abstract 517

Grey P, Johnston M, Petoumenos K et al. Analysis of treatment-associated viral load change during primary HIV infection. Boston: 10th Conference on Retroviruses and Opportunistic Infections, 2003: Abstract 516

Hecht FM, Wang L, Collier A et al. HAART for primary/ early HIV infection associated with improved outcomes after treatment discontinuation? Boston: 10th Conference on Retroviruses and Opportunistic Infections, 2003: Abstract 519

Hermans P, Kabeya K, Clumeck N et al. Successful interruption of antiretroviral therapy (ARVT) in patients with primary HIV infection (PHI). Chicago: 8th Conference on Retroviruses and Opportunistic Infections, 2001: Abstract 290

Hoen B, Fournier I, Charreau I et al. Structured treatment interruptions in primary HIV infection: final results of the multicenter prospective PRIMSTOP pilot trial. San Francisco: 11th Conference on Retroviruses and Opportunistic Infections, 2004: Abstract 395

Kaufmann D, Lichterfeld M, Altfeld M et al. Limited durability of immune control following treated acute HIV infection. San Francisco: 11th Conference on Retroviruses and Opportunistic Infections, 2004: Oral Abstract 24

Kinloch S, Cooper D, Lampe F et al. The QUEST cohort: treatment of primary HIV infection with quadruple HAART: week 48 preliminary results. Boston: 10th Conference on Retroviruses and Opportunistic Infections, 2003: Abstract 520

Lacabaratz-Porret C, Hoen H, Urrutia A et al. Determination of HIV-specific CD8+ and CD4+ responses in structured treatment interruptions in primary HIV infection: results of the multicenter prospective pilot trial PRIMSTOP. San Francisco: 11th Conference on Retroviruses and Opportunistic Infections, 2004: Abstract 396

Lafeuillade A, Counillon E, Poggi C et al. Predictors of plasma HIV RNA control after discontinuation of HAART initiated at acute infection. Boston: 10th Conference on Retroviruses and Opportunistic Infections, 2003: Abstract 513

Lisziewicz J, Rosenberg E, Lieberman J et al. Control of HIV despite the discontinuation of antiretroviral therapy. N Engl J Med 1999; 340: 1683–1684

Lori F, Lewis MG, Xu J et al. Control of SIV rebound through structured treatment interruptions during early infection. Science 2000; 290: 1591–1593

Musey L, Hughes J, Schacker T et al. Cytotoxic T-cell responses, viral load and disease progression in early human immunodeficiency virus type 1 infection. N Engl J Med 1997; 337: 1267–1274

Oxenius A, Price DA, Easterbrook PJ et al. Early highly active antiretroviral therapy for acute HIV-1 infection preserves immune function of CD8+ and CD4+ T lymphocytes. Proc Natl Acad Sci USA 2000; 97: 3382–3387

Rosenberg ES, Altfeld M, Poon SH et al. Immune control of HIV-1 after early treatment of acute infection. Nature 2000; 407: 523–526

Smith D, Grey P, Petoumenos K et al. Virological and immunological predictors of time to initial viral suppression and viral rebound in a randomised trial of combination therapy in primary HIV infection followed by treatment interruption. San Francisco: 11th Conference on Retroviruses and Opportunistic Infections, 2004, Abstract 399

Walker BD, Allen T, Altfeld M et al. Immune control and immune failure in HIV infection. Boston: 10th Conference on Retroviruses and Opportunistic Infections, 2003: Abstract 164

Weintrob A, Giner J, Patrick E, Lennox J, Menezes P, Pilcher C et al. Delayed diagnosis of primary HIV infection after presentation to the health care system. Seattle: 9th Conference on Retroviruses and Opportunistic Infections, 2002: Abstract 360

3.3 Primary HIV Type 1 Infection

H. Jessen

Introduction

Primary HIV infection (PHI) is defined as the time from virus entry to completion of seroconversion. This acute stage of HIV infection is difficult to diagnose – but early diagnosis is important: evidence is emerging that treatment during this phase may alter the course of the disease and may have virological, immunological and clinical benefits. Only sparse controlled findings are available, but the potential benefit of therapy for PHI must be balanced against the known risk of adverse effects of long-term treatment and the development of resistance. Early identification of PHI is also important to prevent unknown transmission of HIV-1 during this period of very high-level viremia.

Immunological and Virological Events during Acute HIV Infection

During primary infection, the HI virus replicates with dramatic speed until the host's immune response can adapt. The plasma viral load often exceeds millions of HIV-1 RNA copies/mL before seroconversion (Rosenberg et al., 2000). During this initial replication cycle, crucial pathogenic mechanisms take place: the virus disseminates into cellular and anatomic sanctuaries and the functional impairment of the immune system starts (Schacker et al., 1996; Schacker et al., 1998). The period of very high viral load lasts only several weeks. During this time, the patient's immune system tries to eradicate the virus, and HIV-1-specific cytotoxic T lymphocytes (CTL) emerge. The formation of HIV-1-specific antibodies marks seroconversion itself, which takes place by week 3–12 after infection (Bush and Satten, 1997).

During seroconversion, the high viral load decreases by several log 10 increments until a steady state is reached where a balance between viral replication and virus-specific immune response limits replication. This viral setpoint is highly predictive for the long-term prognosis (Mellors et al., 1995), and is dependent on the fitness of the virus as well as on genetic factors and immune responses of the host. Patients with the highest setpoints progress most rapidly to AIDS. Before seroconversion, the CD4 cell count sometimes decreases to very low levels and increases again after seroconversion. The count never returns to the value present before HIV infection, and the CD4 cells never regain normal function (Rosenberg et al., 1997; Altfeld et al., 2001).

Genetic factors in the host influence the susceptibility and resistance to HIV infection as well as the velocity of disease progression. A striking mutation is a 32 base-pair deletion in the gene of the chemokine co-receptor CCR5 – called CCR5Δ32 – which is the most important co-receptor for the entry of the virus into the CD4 cell. Homozygous individuals with CCR5Δ32 can be infected only by HIV strains that enter the CD4 cell via the co-receptor CXCR4. Heterozygous individuals have significantly lower viral setpoints and a slower disease progression rate (Michael et al., 1997). The CCR5Δ32 mutation is more prevalent in patients who were known as long-term non-progressors or now as viral controllers. HLA alleles might play a critical role. Others like the "Berlin patient" (Liesziewicz et al., 1999) have not shown specific group characteristics yet.

Clinical Signs and Symptoms

About 40–90% of HIV-infected persons develop symptoms of the "retroviral syndrome", typically 2–4 weeks after infection (Schacker et al., 1996; Kahn and Walker, 1998; Walensky et al., 2001). The symptoms last for 7 to 10 days, rarely longer than 14 days. The retroviral syndrome resembles infectious mononucleosis by Epstein-Barr virus. The symptoms are mostly non-specific and include some of the following: fever, fatigue, pharyngitis, often ulcerative, non-itching rash of the trunk, lymphadenopathy, night sweats, weight loss, myalgia, arthralgia, headache, nausea, vomiting and diarrhea. Single individuals with PHI can show acute renal failure, myocarditis, meningitis, even Guillain-Barré syndrome and, because of a transient low CD4+ cell count, opportunistic infections with *Candida* or *Pneumocystis carinii* can occur. Due to the non-specific nature of the symptoms, only 25% of patients with PHI are diagnosed correctly (Schacker et al., 1996). Patients with more severe, prolonged and persistent symptoms progress more rapidly to AIDS (Keet et al., 1993; Lindback et al., 1994).

Diagnosis

The evaluations needed to diagnose acute HIV-1 infection should be considered if a patient has symptoms of the retroviral syndrome and a history of high-risk exposure, or presents with one or more sexually transmitted diseases. The differential diagnosis should exclude other illnesses such as mononucleosis, CMV infection, hepatitis, influenza, toxoplasmosis, secondary syphilis, systemic lupus erythematosus and drug reaction.

Antibodies have not been formed in very early HIV infection, and serologic tests such as the Western blot do not show a positive result until 22–27 days after acute infection (Busch et al., 1995). HIV infection should be diagnosed by the fourth-generation ELISA test, detecting antibodies, p24 antigen and viral RNA. Most sensitive is the direct measurement of virus RNA with branched chain DNA, PCR and GenProbe, which have a sensitivity of 100% (Hecht et al., 2002). False-positive results can occur in 2–5% of cases. The diagnosis of acute HIV infection must be confirmed with a positive antibody test (Western blot) several weeks later.

Treatment of PHI

Antiretroviral treatment during acute HIV infection may achieve a more effective immune response. Potential benefits include mitigation of acute retroviral symptoms, early prevention of abnormal helper T cell function, decreasing of the initial virus load setpoint, limitation of viral evolution and diversity, and reduction of the risk of transmission at a time of extraordinarily high virus

levels (Kassutto and Rosenberg, 2004). Only few randomized, controlled trials have been conducted in this patient population. The first one compared AZT monotherapy and placebo. The patients who received AZT had fewer opportunistic infections and a greater increase in CD4+ cells (Kinloch-de-Loes et al., 1995). More and more studies – although in only small cohorts – showed that the functional, HIV-1-specific immune response could be enhanced, and that the immune functions of CD8+ and CD4+ T lymphocytes could be preserved with antiretroviral treatment during PHI (Rosenberg et al., 1997; Oxenius et al., 2000; Malhotra et al., 2000; Lacabartz-Porret et al., 2003). A pilot study showed that patients who were treated during PHI and underwent structured treatment interruptions (STI) afterwards had a better immune response (Rosenberg et al., 2000). Most patients were able to stop treatment, and in some the viral setpoint has been <5000 copies/mL for three years. Half of the patients had to start therapy again after a long follow-up interval as the viral load increased again.

When and What?

So far, studies support the use of antiretroviral therapy for PHI, but none have shown a survival benefit. Whether patients with acute HIV infection should be treated and when the treatment should be started remains controversial. Limited durability of viral control following treatment has been shown in a small cohort recently (Kaufmann et al., 2004). The US Department of Health and Human Services (DHHS) recommends considering treatment if the diagnosis is made less than 6 months after infection (US Department of Health and Human Services, 2004). The British HIV Association (BHIVA) recommends treating PHI only for relief of symptoms of acute retroviral syndrome (British HIV Association Guidelines, 2003). And the international AIDS Society (IAS) has no specific recommendations, but refers to the role of STIs in this patient group and recommends using STIs only in the context of a clinical trial (Yeni et al., 2002).

If treatment is considered, it should be a standard triple regime with a protease inhibitor or a non-nucleoside reverse-transcriptase inhibitor. As the virus replicates very fast during PHI, adherence is a critical issue for the success of therapy. Genotype testing can be done and used for additional information, but this testing should not delay therapy. In chronic HIV infection, antiretroviral therapy leads to undetectable viral loads within 8–10 weeks. The time to virus suppression in patients with PHI is not well characterized and differs very widely depending on the virus and immune system. It is not clear if an initial high viral load prolongs the time to virus suppression, or whether an immune system that is still relatively intact and a lower total body virus burden may shorten this time. Once an undetectable viral load is achieved, an STI may be introduced, if possible only in the context of clinical studies. Large randomized trials are urgently needed.

References

Altfeld M, Rosenberg ES, Shankarappa R et al. Cellular immune responses and viral diversity in individuals treated during acute and early HIV-1 infection. J Exp Med 2001; 193: 169–180

British HIV Association Guidelines for the Treatment of HIV Disease with Antiretroviral Therapy, 2003 (accessible under http://www.aidsmap.com/about/bhivagd.asp)

Busch MP, Lee LL, Satten GA et al. Time course of detection of viral and serologic markers preceding human immunodeficiency virus type 1 seroconversion: implications for screening of blood and tissue donors. Transfusion 1995; 35: 91–97

Busch MP, Satten GA. Time course of viremia and antibody seroconversion following human immunodeficiency virus exposure (review). Am J Med 1997; 102: 117–124 (discussion: 125–126)

Hecht FM, Busch MP, Rawal B et al. Use of laboratory tests and clinical symptoms for identification of primary HIV infection. AIDS 2002; 16: 1119–1129

Kahn JO, Walker BD. Acute human immunodeficiency virus type 1 infection. N Engl J Med 1998; 339: 33–39

Kassutto S, Rosenberg ES. Primary HIV type 1 infection. Clin Infect Dis 2004; 38: 1447–1453

Kaufmann DE, Lichterfeld M, Altfeld M et al. Limited durability of viral control following treated acute HIV infection. PLoS Med 2004; 1: e36 (epub ahead of print)

Keet IP, Krijnen P, Koot M et al. Predictors of rapid progression to AIDS in HIV-1 seroconverters. AIDS 1993; 7: 51–57

Kinloch-de-Loes S, Hirschel BJ, Hoen B et al. A controlled trial of zidovudine in primary HIV infection. N Engl J Med 1995; 333: 408–413

Lacabaratz-Porret C, Urrutia A, Doisne JM et al. Impact of antiretroviral therapy and changes in virus load on HIV-specific T cell responses in primary HIV infection. J Infect Dis 2003; 187: 748–757

Liesziewicz J, Rosenberg E, Lieberman J, Jessen H et al. Control of HIV despite the discontinuation of antiretroviral therapy. N Engl J Med 1999; 340: 1683–1684

Lindback S, Brostrom C, Karlsson A, Gaines H. Does symptomatic primary HIV-1 infection accelerate progression to CDC stage IV disease, CD4 count below 200×10^6/L, AIDS and death from AIDS? BMJ 1994; 309: 1535–1537

Malhotra U, Berrey MM, Huang Y et al. Effect of combination antiretroviral therapy on T-cell immunity in acute human immunodeficiency virus type 1 infection. J Infect Dis 2000; 181: 121–131

Mellors JW, Kingsley LA, Rinaldo CR et al. Quantitation of HIV-1 RNA in plasma predicts outcome after seroconversion. Ann Intern Med 1995; 122: 573–579

Michael NL, Chang G, Louie LG et al. The role of viral phenotype and CCR5-gene defects in HIV-1 transmission and disease progression. Nat Med 1997; 3: 338–340

Oxenius A, Price DA, Easterbrook PJ et al. Early highly active antiretroviral therapy for acute HIV-1 infection preserves immune function of CD8$^+$ and CD4$^+$ T lymphocytes. Proc Natl Acad Sci USA 2000; 97: 3382–3387

Rosenberg ES, Billingsley JM, Caliendo AM et al. Vigorous HIV-1 specific CD4$^+$ T cell responses associated with control of viremia. Science 1997; 278: 1447–1450

Rosenberg ES, Altfeld M, Poon SH et al. Immune control of HIV-1 after early treatment of acute infection. Nature 2000; 407: 523–526

Schacker T, Collier AC, Hughes J, Shea T, Corey L. Clinical and epidemiologic features of primary HIV infection. Ann Intern Med 1996; 125: 257–264 (erratum in: Ann Intern Med 1997; 126: 174)

Schacker T, Hughes JP, Shea T, Coombs R, Corey L. Biological and virologic characteristics of primary HIV infection. Ann Intern Med 1998; 128: 613–620

US Department of Health and Human Services Panel on Clinical Practise for Treatment of HIV Infection. Guidelines for the use of antiretroviral agents in HIV-1 infected adults and adolescents, 2004 available under http://www.aidsinfo.nih.gov.

Walensky RP, Rosenberg ES, Ferraro MJ, Losina E, Walker BD, Freedberg KA. Investigation of primary human immunodeficiency virus infection in patients who test positive for heterophile antibody. Clin Infect Dis 2001; 33: 570–572

Yeni PG, Hammer SM, Carpenter CC et al. Antiretroviral treatment for adult HIV infection in 2002: updated recommendations of the international AIDS Society – USA panel. JAMA 2002; 288: 222–235

Index

A

abacavir   27, 32
Ac-DAG   71
  CD4 cell counts   73
  cohort   72
  inclusion criteria   71
  initial viral load   73
  mean changes in CD4 cell
  count   75
  results   72
acute HIV infection
  immunization studies   50
  immunological events   78
  supervised treatment
  interruptions   36 ff
  symptoms   70
  virological events   78
acute HIV-1 infection
  differential diagnosis   79
  treatment   79
  triple regime   79
acute retroviral
syndrome   72
  CD4 cell count   73
  viral load   73
acute viral syndrome   1
ADARC   50
adenovirus type 5 vector   22
AIDS
  immune-based
  therapies   21 ff
AIEDRP AI502   50
aldrithiol-2   24
ALVAC   23
ALVAC vCP1452   50
amprenavir   33
analytic treatment
interruptions   52
antibodies
  escaping   12
  neutralizing   12

antigen processing
mutations   16
antiretroviral drugs   60
  development of HIV
  resistance   60
arthralgia   79
autoimmunity   27
autologous vaccination   50
  results   50
autovaccination   24
AZT   79

B

Berlin patient   69

C

canarypox   47
Candida esophagitis   70
carbovir triphosphate   27
CATCH study   66
  baseline resistance   66
CCR7 T cells   2
CD4 T cells   1
  CMV-specific   2
    functional signature   2 f
    phenotypic signature   2 f
  count   75
    mean changes   75
  HIV-1-specific   1
    functional characteri-
    zation   1
  progressive depletion   2
  untreated patients   53
    absolute counts   53
CD4⁺+ T cells
  effect of treatment
  interruption   38
CD8 T cells   5
  HIV-1-specific   1
  untreated patients
    absolute counts   53

CD8⁺+ T cells   5
  HIV-1-specific   5 ff
    responses in HIV-1
    infection   5 ff
CellCept™   28
cellular immunity   21
central memory [T$_{CM}$]   2
chronic infection   47 f
  immunization trials   47
  therapeutic studies   48 f
clinical epidemiology   60 ff
clinical management   60 ff
CMV infection   79
compartmentalization   61
cyclosporin   29
cytokine-augmented DNA
vaccines   21
cytomegalovirus (CMV)
infection   1

D

dendritic cell-based
immunization   23
dendritic cell-targeted
immunization   25
  mechanism of action   25
Dermavir   25
diarrhea   70, 79
didanosine   27
direct targeted dendritic cell
topical immunization   24
disease progression   15, 62
  consequences of transmitted
  resistance   62
  impact of HIV-1
  sequence   15
DNA prime/viral vector boost
strategy   22
drug reaction   79
drug resistance   60 ff
  transmitted   63

E

effector memory [T$_{EM}$]   2
ELISPOT   53
endoplasmatic reticulum   16
Env   6
    structural HIV-1 protein   6
env/gag plasmid DNA
vaccine   22
envelope glycoprotein
gp120   21
epidemiology   65
ER-resident amino-
peptidase   16
escape mutations
    reversion   16
    transmission   16
ex vivo dendritic cell-based
immunization   24
exanthema   70

F

fatigue   79
fever   70, 79
fidelity
    definition   60
fitness   60 ff
    definition   60
    transmission   63

G

Gag   6
    structural HIV-1 protein   6
genetic barrier   60
    definition   60
genetic plasticity   5
    HIV-1 virus   5
genotype
    definition   60
genotypic assays   62
genotyping
    diagnosis of resistance   62
gp120   21

H

HAART   5, 21, 32 ff, 36, 60
    failing   61
    pregnancy   64
    results   33
headache   79
hepatitis   79

heterologous prime-boost
strategy   22
highly active antiretroviral
therapy
    see HAART
HIV
    envelope subunits   47
    fitness   61
    genetic diversity   61
    immune-based thera-
    py   21 ff
    infection
        acute
            pathways   45
            supervised treatment
            interruptions   36 ff
            symptoms   70
            treatment strategies
            70
        primary
            management in
            Germany   69 ff
            mechanisms of
            resistance   61
    lipopeptide vaccines   23
HIV resistance
    transmission   66
HIV-1
    early treatment   4
    Gag protein sequence   13
    immune control
        impact of viral sequence
        evolution   12 ff
    infection
        acute
            HIV-1-specific CD8$^+$+ T
            cells
        primary   1
    replication dynamics   12
    RNA replication   32
        long-term control   32 ff
    sequence
        diversity   12
        impact on disease
        progression   15
    subtypes   62
        non-B subtypes   63
        subtype B   62
    virus   5
        sequence variations   5
        world-wide spread   5
HIV-1-specific CD4 T cells   1
    functional characteri-
    zation   1

functional signature   2 f
    phenotypic signature   2 f
HIV-1-specific CD8 T cells   1
HIV-1-specific CD8$^+$+ T
cells   5 ff
    responses in HIV-1
    infection   5 ff
HLA class 1
    alleles   8
    genetic background   8
hydroxyurea   26 ff
    mechanisms of action   27
    myeloproliferative
    disorders   27
    sickle-cell anemia   27

I

IL-2   28
    mechanism of action   28
IL-2-augmented DNA   22
immune boosting   36
immune evasion   12
    alternative mechanism   16
immune function
    paradoxical restoration   27
immune modulators   21, 26
immune response
    cellular   12
    humoral   12
    innate component   45
immunization
    dendritic cell-based   23
        ex vivo   24
    trials
        chronic infection   47
    studies
        acute infection   50
        therapeutic
            future concerns   52
Immunogen   47
immunology
    acute HIV infection   44
influenza   79
innate immunization   46
inosine monophosphate
dehydrogenase   28
intracellular cytokine
staining   53

L

lamivudine   70
lipopeptides   47

long-term non-progressors (LTNP)   1
lopinavir   70
lymphadenopathy   70, 79
lymphocyte function
  impairment   26

M

modified vaccinia Ankara (MVA) vector   22
mononucleosis   79
mother-to-child transmission   64
mutations   62
myalgia   79
mycophenolate mofetil   28
  therapy   32 ff
mycophenolic acid (MPA)   26, 28, 32
  effect on cell activation   32
  effect on HIV-1 infection   32
  mechanism of action   28

N

nausea   79
NCHECR study   51
Nef
  HIV-1 gene product   6
neutralizing antibodies   46
nevirapine   64
night sweats   79
non-nucleoside reverse transcriptase inhibitors (NNRTIs)   61
nucleoside-analogue reverse transcriptase inhibitors (NRTIs)   60

P

pharyngitis   70, 79
phenotype
  definition   60
phenotypic assays   62
phenotyping
  diagnosis of resistance   62
PHI (primary HIV infection)
  immunology   44
  therapeutic vaccination   44 ff
Pol
  structural HIV-1 protein   6
polymerase chain reaction   62

post-exposure prophylaxis   64
pregnancy
  HAART   64
primary HIV infection (PHI)
  management in Germany   69 ff
  when to start therapy   32
primary HIV-1 infection   1, 78
  clinical signs   78 f
  definition   78
  diagnosis   79
  symptoms   78
primary mutation
  definition   60
primary resistance mutation
  definition   60
primary resistance   60
Prime-DAG   70
  CD4 cell counts   73
    mean changes   75
  inclusion criteria   70
  initial viral load   73
  mean changes in absolute CD4 cell count   72
  mean changes in viral load   71
  results   70, 72
  cohort   70
prophylaxis
  post-exposure   64
protease inhibitors   61
PRPP synthetase   28
public health impact   65
PULSE   50
purines
  general synthesis scheme   26

Q

Quest study   50 f
quick replication   61

R

rapamycin (RAPA)   28
  mechanism of action   28
rash
  ulcerative, non-itching of trunk   79
recombinant gp160   50
REMUNE   47
renal transplant rejection
  mycophenolic acid   28

rapamycin   28
replication
  dynamics   12
  infidelity   61
resistance   60
  diagnosis   62
    genotyping   62
    phenotyping   62
  HIV   61
    mechanisms   61
  transmission   60 ff
    risk groups   64
  transmitted   62
    consequences for disease progression   62
    therapeutic consequences   62
retroviral syndrome   78
Rev
  HIV-1 gene product   6
reversion to wild type   63
Rhesus macaque
  immune responses to HIV   22 f
ribonucleotide reductase   28
ritonavir   70

S

sanctuary sites   62
secondary mutation
  definition   60
secondary resistance mutation
  definition   60
secondary syphilis   79
seroconversion   7
sexually transmitted diseases   79
SIV-specific memory T cells (SMTC)   24
SPARTAC   50
SPREAD program   66
stavudine   33
stomatitis   70
structured treatment interruptions   50
  results   50
structured/supervised treatment interruption   32
supervised treatment interruption
  acute HIV infection   36 ff
  evolution of CD4$^+$+ T cell count   38

evolution of viral load   38
period of viral control
achieved   37
time to failure   37
unique   33
results   33
synergism
abacavir and amprenavir   33
abacavir and mycophenolic
acid   32
system lupus erythematosus 79

T

Tat
HIV-1 gene product   6
therapeutic vaccine
strategies   21
tonsillitis   70
toxoplasmosis   79
transmission
fitness   63
mother-to-child   64
resistance
measurements   65
risk groups   64
role of PHI   63
of resistant viruses   60
of resistance   60 ff
transmitted drug
resistance   63
transmitted resistance   62
consequences for disease
progression   62
therapeutic consequences
62
trunk
ulcerative, non-itching
rash   79

U

unique supervised treatment
interruption   33
results   33

UNITEMORE study   66
untreated patients
absolute CD4 counts   53
absolute CD8 counts   53
CD4 cell count   76
viral load   76

V

vaccination
therapeutic
in PHI   44 ff
vaccines   21
candidates   47
avian pox viruses
alone   47
in combination with
envelope subunits   47
DNA constructs   47
inactivated virus with
envelope components
removed   47
subunits of HIV
envelope   47
cytokine-augmented
DNA   21
DC-targeted   22
DNA   22
ex vivo dendritic
cell-based   22
lipopeptide   22
preventative   21
therapeutic   21
efficacy   21
laboratory assess-
ment   52 f
vertical transmission   46, 64
Vif
accessory HIV-1 protein   6
viral evolution
driving forces   17
viral load
decline   14
mean changes during
treatment   74

viral protein
kinetics of expression   6
viral reverse transcriptase   12
viral sequence evolution
impact on immune control
of HIV-1   12 ff
viremia   39
duration   39
correlation with clinical
markers   39
correlation with genetic
markers   39
relation to HIV-1-specific T
cell response   39
peak   14
virostatics   21, 26
virus-like particles   47
vomiting   79
Vpr
accessory HIV-1 protein   6
Vpu
accessory HIV-1 protein   6

W

WATCH study   66
weight loss   79
wild type
reversion to   63

Z

zidovudine   33, 64, 70